HEALTH SYSTEMS SCIENCE EDUCATION

DEVELOPMENT and IMPLEMENTATION

The AMA MedEd Innovation Series

The Master Adaptive Learner
Edited by William B. Cutrer, Martin V. Pusic, Larry D. Gruppen, Maya M. Hammoud, and Sally A. Santen

Value-Added Roles for Medical Students
Edited by Jed Gonzalo, Maya M. Hammoud, and Gregory W. Schneider

Coaching in Medical Education
Edited by Maya M. Hammoud, Nicole M. Deiorio, Margaret Moore, and Margaret Wolff

Health Systems Science Implementation: Development and Implementation
Edited by Rosalyn Maben-Feaster, Maya M. Hammoud, Jeffrey Borkan, Ami DeWaters, Jed Gonzalo, and Stephanie R. Starr

HEALTH SYSTEMS SCIENCE EDUCATION

DEVELOPMENT and IMPLEMENTATION

The AMA MedEd Innovation Series

ROSALYN MABEN-FEASTER, MD, MPH
University of Michigan Medical School

MAYA M. HAMMOUD, MD, MBA
University of Michigan Medical School
American Medical Association

JEFFREY BORKAN, MD, PhD
The Warren Alpert Medical School, Brown University

AMI DEWATERS, MSc, MD
Penn State Medical Center

JED GONZALO, MSc, MD
Penn State Medical Center

STEPHANIE STARR, MD
Mayo Clinic Alix School of Medicine

ELSEVIER

Elsevier
1600 John F. Kennedy Blvd.
Ste 1800
Philadelphia, PA 19103-2899

Notice

Practitioners and researchers must always rely on their own experience and knowledge in evaluating and using any information, methods, compounds or experiments described herein. Because of rapid advances in the medical sciences, in particular, independent verification of diagnoses and drug dosages should be made. To the fullest extent of the law, no responsibility is assumed by Elsevier, authors, editors or contributors for any injury and/or damage to persons or property as a matter of products liability, negligence or otherwise, or from any use or operation of any methods, products, instructions, or ideas contained in the material herein.

Content Strategist: Elyse W. O'Grady
Content Development Specialist: Nicole Congleton
Publishing Services Manager: Shereen Jameel
Project Manager: Maria Shalini
Design Direction: Patrick C. Ferguson

Printed in the United States of America

Last digit is the print number: 9 8 7 6 5 4 3 2 1

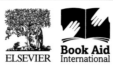

Working together to grow libraries in developing countries

www.elsevier.com • www.bookaid.org

CONTRIBUTORS

Nana E. Coleman, MD, EdM
Baylor College of Medicine
Houston, Texas
Chapter 1

Susan A. DeRiemer, PhD
Meharry Medical College
Nashville, Tennessee
Chapter 6

Mitchell J. Gitkind, MD
UMass Chan Medical School
Worcester, Massachusetts
Chapter 1

Jed Gonzalo, MSc, MD
Penn State College of Medicine
Hershey, Pennsylvania
Chapter 2

Ronan Hallowell, EdD
Keck School of Medicine of University of Southern
    California
Los Angeles, California
Chapter 7

Maya M. Hammoud, MD, MBA
University of Michigan Medical School
Ann Arbor, Michigan;
American Medical Association
Chicago, Illinois
Chapter 2

Lisanne Hauck, MD, MSEd
CUNY School of Medicine
New York City, New York
Chapter 6

Beth A. Hawks, PhD, MHA*
Uniformed Services University of the Health Sciences
    School of Medicine
Bethesda, Maryland
Chapter 7

Tracey L. Henry, MD, MPH, MS
Emory University School of Medicine
Atlanta, Georgia
Chapter 5

Jung G. Kim, MPH, PhD
Kaiser Permanente Bernard J. Tyson
School of Medicine
Pasadena, California
Chapter 1

Kimberly D. Lomis, MD
American Medical Association
Chicago, Illinois
Chapter 2

Jennifer Meka, PhD, MSEd
Jacobs School of Medicine and Biomedical Sciences
University at Buffalo
Buffalo, New York
Chapter 3

Rani Nandiwada, MD, MS
Penn State College of Medicine
Hershey, Pennsylvania
Chapter 4

Daniel A. Novak, PhD
University of California, Riverside
School of Medicine
Riverside, California
Chapter 7

* The contents, views, or opinions expressed in this publication or presentation are those of the authors and do not necessarily reflect official policy or position of Uniformed Services University of the Health Sciences, the Department of Defense, or Departments of the Army, Navy, or Air Force. Mention of trade names, commercial products, or organizations does not imply endorsement by the United States Government.

Casey Olm-Shipman, MD, MS
University of North Carolina School of Medicine
Chapel Hill, North Carolina
Chapter 5

Dharmini Shah Pandya, MD
Lewis Katz School of Medicine at Temple University
Philadelphia, Pennsylvania
Chapter 5

Dimitrios Papanagnou, MD, MPH, EdD(c)
Sidney Kimmel Medical College at Thomas Jefferson
    University
Philadelphia, Pennsylvania
Chapter 4

Valerie G. Press, MD, MPH
University of Chicago Medicine
Chicago, Illinois
Chapter 6

F. Lee Revere, PhD
University of Florida
Gainesville, Florida
Chapter 7

Rachel Marie E. Salas, MD, MEd
Johns Hopkins University School of Medicine
Baltimore, Maryland
Chapter 6

Sally A. Santen, MD, PhD
Virginia Commonwealth University
School of Medicine
Richmond, Virginia;
University of Cincinnati College of Medicine
Cincinnati, Ohio;
American Medical Association
Chicago, Illinois
Chapter 2

Karen E. Segerson, MD
University of Washington
Seattle, Washington
Chapter 3

Shirin Shafazand, MD, MS
University of Miami Miller School of Medicine
Miami, Florida
Chapter 4

Meredith Volle, MD, MPH
Southern Illinois University School of Medicine
Springfield, Illinois
Chapter 4

Paul F. Weber, MD, RPh, MBA
Rutgers Robert Wood Johnson Medical School
New Brunswick, New Jersey
Chapter 1

Peter Weir, MD, MPH
University of Utah
Salt Lake City, Utah
Chapter 3

Earla J. White, PhD, MEd
A.T. Still University–School of Osteopathic
Medicine in Arizona
Mesa, Arizona
Chapter 3

FOREWORD

The American Medical Association's (AMA's) Accelerating Change in Medical Education Consortium creates new approaches to health professions training to ultimately improve patient outcomes. Our Consortium has produced innovations in a number of areas that are being adopted across many schools. To enhance the dissemination of these innovations, we are excited to present a series of books for their adoption at additional health professions schools and training programs.

The AMA MedEd Innovation Series provides practical guidance for local implementation of the education innovations from the AMA Consortium. This book on implementing health systems science into the medical education curriculum is the fourth in our AMA series. Future subjects will include improving change management for faculty and incorporating the electronic health record into curricula.

Health Systems Science Education: Development and Implementation presents the work of experts across the country who have implemented health systems science in undergraduate and graduate medical education. As the field of health systems science continues to grow, we hope you find this book to be a valuable resource in your curriculum.

We are pleased to offer this fourth book in the AMA MedEd Innovation Series and look forward to learning about your experiences in implementing health systems science at your institution.

Sanjay V. Desai, MD
Chief Academic Officer
American Medical Association

ACKNOWLEDGMENTS

The editors and authors of this book would like to thank Sarah Ayala of the American Medical Association (AMA) for her project management. Without her, this book would not exist. We'd also like to thank Amanda Moutrage, also of the AMA, for her scheduling skills and project assistance. Victoria Stagg Elliott, AMA, gets our thanks for her copyediting and catching our misspellings and misused words. Kevin Heckman of the AMA and project manager of the AMA MedEd Innovation Series gets our gratitude for his support of this book. We give additional thanks to the members of the AMA Accelerating Change in Medical Education Consortium who contributed to this book's creation, and to Sanjay V. Desai, MD, the AMA's Group Vice President for medical education. Without his leadership, this book would not have been possible.

CONTENTS

1. Getting Started: General Considerations for Health Systems Science Implementation, **1**
   Jung G. Kim, Mitchell J. Gitkind, Nana E. Coleman, and Paul F. Weber

2. Health Systems Science Competencies in Medical Education, **19**
   Jed Gonzalo, Sally A. Santen, Kimberly D. Lomis, and Maya M. Hammoud

3. Health Systems Science Implementation in Pre-clerkship Curricula, **35**
   Karen E. Segerson, Peter Weir, Earla J. White, and Jennifer Meka

4. Health Systems Science Implementation in the Clinical Learning Environment: Undergraduate Medical Education, **51**
   Dimitrios Papanagnou, Shirin Shafazand, Meredith Volle, and Rani Nandiwada

5. Health Systems Science Implementation in Graduate Medical Education, **65**
   Casey Olm-Shipman, Tracey L. Henry, and Dharmini Shah Pandya

6. The Role of Interprofessional Education and Collaborative Practice in Health Systems Science Curricula, **85**
   Rachel Marie E. Salas, Lisanne Hauck, Susan A. DeRiemer, and Valerie G. Press

7. Sustainability in a Health Systems Science Program: Assessment, Evaluation, and Continuous Improvement, **103**
   Daniel A. Novak, Beth A. Hawks, F. Lee Revere, and Ronan Hallowell

Glossary, 119

Index, 123

xi

Getting Started: General Considerations for Health Systems Science Implementation

Jung G. Kim, Mitchell J. Gitkind, Nana E. Coleman, and Paul F. Weber

CHAPTER OUTLINE

Chapter Summary, 1
Introduction, 2
Overview: Phases of Curricular Transformation, 2
What Is Health Systems Science?, 3
Where to Begin With a Health System Science
   Curriculum?, 4
   Establish a Sense of Urgency, 5
   Create a Guiding Coalition, 5
   Develop a Shared Vision and Strategy, 7
Building Highly Effective Teams for Health Systems
   Science Implementation, 8
   Why Teamwork?, 8
   What Does the Ideal Team Look Like?, 8
   How Do We Attract the Right Team Members?, 11

How Do Teams Work Best Among Themselves and
   With Others?, 12
What Is the Intersection Between Systems Thinking,
   Team Science, and Health Systems Science?, 12
Strategies to Maximize Team Effectiveness, 12
Evaluating the Current State: Educator Competency,
   Curricular Structure, and the Learning Environment, 14
   Educator Competency, 14
   Curricular Structure, 14
   The Learning Environment, 15
Completing the Pre-implementation Process, 16
Conclusion, 16
Take-Home Points, 16
Questions for Further Thought, 16

CHAPTER SUMMARY

Medical education must be agile to align with complex and dynamic learning environments and health care delivery systems that are coupled with the heightened societal expectations on the physician workforce. Reimagining curriculum in undergraduate, graduate, and continuing medical education ushers in the opportunity to insert health systems science (HSS), the third pillar of medical education, that can teach how care is delivered, how health professionals work together to deliver that care, and how the health system can improve patient care and health care delivery.

The successful implementation of HSS curriculum requires purposeful strategies via effective change management practices that integrate organizational assets, engage stakeholders, and mobilize a highly effective team. Pre-implementation is a vital stage that antecedes the implementation process to promote successful outcomes. This stage includes mapping the current state via performing a needs assessment for curricular transformation, incorporating best practices for change management processes, gauging stakeholder readiness and state of change followed by stakeholder identification, and appreciating the attributes of highly effective teams. As medical educators complete the pre-implementation stage, defining shared success and roadmapping the team's journey are prerequisites to ensuring that an HSS curriculum implementation is fully achieved.

INTRODUCTION

> *"Transformation is a process, not an event."*
> —*John P. Kotter[1]*

In complex and dynamic learning environments, medical education must remain agile so it can meet evolving health care delivery needs and the heightened societal expectations on the physician workforce. Factors such as new and emerging diseases (e.g., COVID-19), rapid scientific and therapeutic advances, and enhanced standards that underlie medical education across its continuum have required educators to reimagine their approach to undergraduate, graduate, and continuing medical education. Consequently, a reexamination of current curricular content and assessment standards reveals opportunities to infuse HSS topics throughout the educational process. As an affirmation of the need and importance of reexamination, reports across US medical schools reveal curricular change is prevalent. For medical schools reporting to the Association of American Medical College's (AAMC) Curriculum Inventory Report, nearly 81% of schools have reported a change in their curriculum in the past 3 years, with 35% of schools in the planning stage or implementing change in the near future. Furthermore, almost one-third of schools have begun implementation.[2]

Momentum and interest to teach and assess the importance for health professionals to be systems based in their responses in the health care delivery system have built exponentially and globally. Over the past decades, the culmination for the demand of systems-based medical education has illuminated the importance of integrating HSS into the curriculum of health professions schools, postgraduate training, and continuing education programs. For individuals and teams embarking on the implementation of any curricular change endeavor, it is essential for them to initially include a **pre-implementation** stage. This permits a more holistic view of the challenges and requirements of

curriculum implementation, and identifies targeted strategies that address potential challenges at the onset of curriculum change. Pre-implementation planning has demonstrated a marked increase for the chance of implementation success. In organizations where process and information flows have been critically observed, nearly 70% of projects fail during implementation when a rigorous pre-implementation stage is bypassed.[3]

OVERVIEW: PHASES OF CURRICULAR TRANSFORMATION

The pre-implementation stage ignites a series of steps as part of curriculum development and managing change within an institution. Fig. 1.1 describes a synthesized conceptual model relevant to curriculum transformation that integrates the Kotter change management process with the Kern curriculum development model.[4] The model outlines the following two phases that will determine the extent of the curriculum change process.

The following guiding questions encompass the initial vision and planning phases during the pre-implementation stage:

- Is the institution in the initial vision and planning phase and considering the role of HSS core domains in the curriculum and/or the institution at large?
- Has the vision been decided that HSS core domains should be adopted into the curriculum, yet curriculum designers are planning out the resources and processes to proceed?

For example, in the initial vision phase, an institution may be still considering the **value-added** drivers of HSS core domains and the magnitude of change needed to their curriculum. These drivers require a more involved effort of organizational **assets** and **stakeholders** depending on the magnitude of change. If the institution already has a firm sense of its vision, strategy, and objectives with HSS-related content, curriculum developers can build on available organizational assets and stakeholders, requiring less formal planning during the pre-implementation stage. Establishing these pre-implementation initial steps lays the foundation to the curricular change management process. As the vision and planning phase concludes, curriculum change proceeds into the implementation and maintenance phase, as discussed in the subsequent chapters.

This chapter focuses on the necessary aspects of the pre-implementation stage to recognize the value-added drivers of HSS, including identifying key assets, engaging key stakeholders, creating a shared vision, building consensus, and deploying a highly effective team to implement HSS curriculum and related initiatives iteratively and longitudinally.

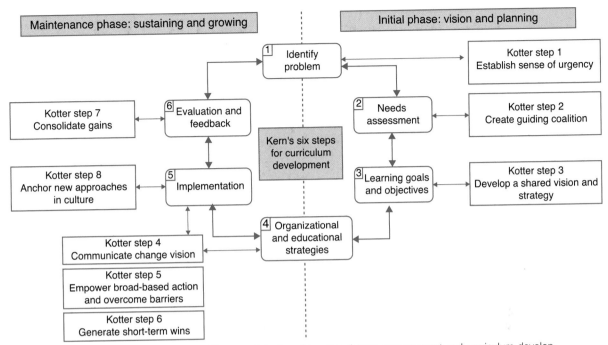

Fig. 1.1 Synthesized Kotter and Kern models describing the change management and curriculum development processes. (Reprinted with permission from Gonzalo JD, Lucey C, Wolpaw T, Chang A. Value-added clinical systems learning roles for medical students that transform education and health: a guide for building partnerships between medical schools and health systems. *Acad Med.* 2017;92(5):602.)

WHAT IS HEALTH SYSTEMS SCIENCE?

In response to the calls to evolve medical education, the American Medical Association (AMA) launched the Accelerating Change in Medical Education Consortium in 2013. One significant contribution of the AMA's initiative has been the framing and description of HSS as a third pillar of medical education.[3] HSS builds on the foundational efforts in systems-based practice (SBP), patient safety, quality improvement, and population health.[3,5] Characterized as "how health care is delivered to, and received by, patients, and populations," HSS teaches a deeper understanding of the health care delivery culture and environment, inclusive of the multitude of settings that culminate into the systems in which patients receive care and health care professionals practice.[3,6] In addition to training health care professionals about systems of care embedded in traditional medical settings, HSS catalyzes medical education to address root causes of health inequities and better assimilate upstream health systems science topics, including but not limited to the social determinants of health, health equity, advocacy, and addressing disparities across society.[3,7,8]

As illustrated in Fig. 1.2, HSS encompasses core functional domains, foundational domains, and a linking domain (**systems thinking**) that define its curricular content and scope of practice.[3] In parallel with the AMA-based initiatives, medical education organizations, including the AAMC and the Accreditation Council for Graduate Medical Education (ACGME), have increasingly encouraged inclusion of HSS content across the educational continuum.[9,10] AAMC has developed a robust set of quality improvement and patient safety (QIPS) competencies that extend beyond the undergraduate medical education (UME) and graduate medical education (GME) levels to include faculty development.[9] ACGME's focus includes the Clinical Learning Environment Review (CLER) Program and its harmonized Milestones (Milestones 2.0) to assess for the core physician competencies, including SBP, toward unsupervised practice.[10,11] As these key stakeholders continue to socialize the importance of HSS, the heart of why HSS continues to proliferate is to evolve educational programs that serve as the critical driver of physician identity formation. This formation must include societal demands on physicians to be inclusive in a community of practice. In this manner, physicians serve as **systems citizens** who can respond beyond the traditional one-on-one patient-to-physician encounter and operate independently within a larger context beyond the walls of the health care delivery

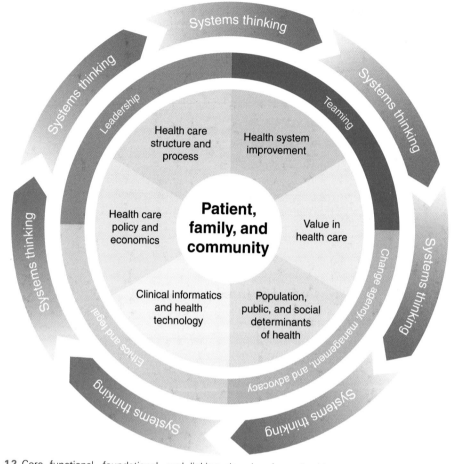

Fig. 1.2 Core functional, foundational, and linking domains for a health systems science curriculum. (Reprinted with permission of the American Medical Association. ©Copyright American Medical Association 2020. All rights reserved.)

system.[5,7] Systems citizenship expands the physician's role to reflect this obligation to society, going beyond altruism and compassion and creating a synergistic relationship with the health care delivery system—all to improve patient and population health.

Health systems science is taught, practiced, and learned in multiple settings, including classrooms and the clinical environment.[4,5] Clerkships, ambulatory continuity clinics, inpatient hospital rounding, and even quality improvement meetings all embody HSS. In these settings, learners are exposed to the knowledge, skills, and behavioral attitudes that manifest to the systems-based core competencies and educational outcomes that medical education and society expect of the physician profession. Organizationally, the learning environment entails "systems of care" consisting of interdependent components that provide education to

learners, and health care to patients with the goal to heal and improve their outcomes.[12] As learners are immersed into these systems, identifying the core concepts to teach within these systems of care is an essential task for pre-implementing HSS curriculum.[5] As learners progress through the stages of learning HSS concepts, their professional identity as systems citizens is crystallized. When achieved, systems citizens will serve as ambassadors to guide others who co-reside in their learning environment.

WHERE TO BEGIN WITH A HEALTH SYSTEMS SCIENCE CURRICULUM?

Transformation of any curriculum must consider effective change management practices that consider the principles of sustainable **scale** and successful **spread** across an institution.

As described in Fig. 1.1, the Kotter change management process integrated with the Kern curriculum development model outlines the following steps that scaffold on each other to accelerate and sustain change:

1. **Establish a sense of urgency:** What is the window of opportunity that is open?
2. **Create a guiding coalition:** Who are the stakeholders, visible or not, who can accelerate the process?
3. **Develop a shared vision and strategies:** What is the North Star or goal that speaks to stakeholders?
4. **Communicate the change vision:** How can you communicate the goals to all stakeholders in an effective and persuasive way?
5. **Empower broad-based action and overcome barriers:** How have past opportunities fallen through, and what prevented them from flourishing?
6. **Generate short-term wins:** How can one build small successes early and often to create momentum?
7. **Consolidate gains:** How can one maintain momentum to scale and spread across an institution?
8. **Anchor new approaches in culture:** How can one foster a new culture from the change to ensure changes are sustainable?

This chapter focuses on the first three steps of this model as well as the importance of building effective teams. The implementation chapters focus on steps 4 to 6, and the last chapter applies steps 7 and 8 for program sustainability and continuous quality improvement.

Establish a Sense of Urgency

The foundational step to the pre-implementation curricular transformation process is to establish a sense of urgency for change. The value to implementing HSS curriculum underscores the following statistics reflective of the US health care delivery system:

- US health outcomes include the highest infant mortality rates and the highest obesity rates among all high-income countries globally.[13,14]
- The United States spends nearly 18% of its gross domestic product on health care resources, more than any nation in the world.[15]
- Twenty-eight million Americans are uninsured, limiting their access to health care.[16]
- Ten percent of patients are harmed by preventable medical errors.[17]
- Forty-two percent of physicians report practice burnout, with common factors cited as excessive bureaucratic tasks and lack of work–life balance.[18]

These systems-related drivers inform national health reform efforts that demand a physician workforce that can demonstrate the necessary readiness and resiliently respond to these complex challenges accordingly. The drivers and values for implementing HSS curriculum highlight the realities with operationalizing medical education embedded in health care delivery systems. Factors related to best preparing health professions students, trainees, and workforce professionals who are responsive to patients, their families, and communities at large amplify the value for teaching and assessing HSS and related systems-based educational outcomes.[19]

Illuminating and incorporating specific drivers and values to align curriculum with the health care delivery system is key to building a sense of urgency to catalyze the curriculum change process. As the sense of urgency is established, proceeding with the subsequent steps of the change management process hinges next on creating a guiding coalition that includes engaging stakeholders and creating a shared vision.

Create a Guiding Coalition

Stakeholders are generally defined as persons, groups, or institutions with a vested interest for organizational strategies that may impact them.[20] They contribute their priorities, constraints, and questions. These elements triangulate, whether or not there is a legitimate institutional urgency for change, while creating complexity in the change management process. Identifying and evaluating stakeholders are key steps in recognizing and preparing to engage them that are critical to the curriculum transformation process. Identifying stakeholders could build from the evaluation of the institution's existing and associated assets as described in the current state needs assessments. These stakeholders could include, but are not limited to, individuals across the medical education continuum ranging from internal to external leadership to front-line individuals. Examples may include students, residents, faculty, instructional designers, and health care professional teams. In addition, stakeholders with authority and oversight could comprise of members at the chair or decanal level, designated institutional officers, service-line chiefs, and even accreditors. Furthermore, stakeholders who support or even challenge the implementation process can provide a balanced perspective to any curricular transformation. Proceeding without recognizing their institution's key stakeholders and incorporating these stakeholders' respective readiness for change opens the door for implementation challenges, obstacles, and failure.

Organizational assets are not stand-alone resources simply available to procure at will. As with any system with interdependencies, assets are linked to a network of stakeholders who have a vested interest in them and bring authority, credibility, and advocacy to the change management process.[20,21] Unveiling stakeholders who may be "hidden" or distal to everyday curriculum operations will provide a clearer understanding of the impact of curricular transformation and maintain the inertia of change management.

The following worksheet adapted from the Centers for Disease Control and Prevention (CDC) participatory model operationalizes the process of stakeholder engagement through two parts: a stakeholder analysis and an engagement plan.[20] A stakeholder analysis (Table 1.1) includes identifying a stakeholder, how much they will be impacted by the curricular transformation, and their level of involvement, and identifying their priorities and constraints in accordance with their role in the institution.

Using a chair of an academic department as an example of a stakeholder, Table 1.1 outlines a path for stakeholder engagement, starting with stakeholder analysis. Although a department chair may not directly write and teach HSS curriculum, this person holds a key stake in implementing the curriculum via resource allocation, such as financial and faculty resources.

Table 1.2 maps out an engagement plan, including reviewing the list of stakeholders as depicted in Table 1.1,

sorting them by categories that are contingent on the overall phase of change for curriculum transformation identified in the previous section. These categories consider the role of the stakeholder, ranging from operational to advocate. A checklist of questions that stakeholders may ask includes: Who will benefit from the curriculum transformation (utility)? How much time and effort are needed (feasibility)? Is the curricular area selected appropriate to transform (propriety)? Have we considered all relevant stakeholders (accuracy)?

A checklist of questions for stakeholders during the engagement plan includes:
- **Utility:** Who will benefit from the curriculum transformation?
- **Feasibility:** How much time and effort are needed?
- **Propriety:** Is the curricular area selected appropriate to transform?
- **Accuracy:** Have we considered all relevant stakeholders?

A key concept that underscores stakeholder engagement is a stakeholder's readiness for change. The commitment to change is dependent on a stakeholder's state of readiness, which impacts their receptivity for innovation,

TABLE 1.1 Stakeholder Analysis Template

Stakeholder	How Are They Impacted by the Curricular Transformation?	What Level of Involvement Do They Have in Curriculum Implementation?	What Are the Priorities Most Meaningful to Them Based on Their Job Role?	What Are Their Most Significant Constraints Based on Their Job Role?
Example: chair of academic department	Accountability to dean, alignment with department's charter	Accountable for course directors, faculty	Meeting departmental budget and accreditation standards	Allocation of resources equitably and standardization of processes

TABLE 1.2 Stakeholder Engagement Template

At what phase of change is the curriculum transformation? (Exploration? Decision and planning? Implementation? Maintenance and continuous improvement?)
Which of the stakeholders are central to the operational components of the curriculum?
Which of the stakeholders above will increase the credibility of the curriculum?
Which of the stakeholders above will advocate changes institutionally?
Which of the stakeholders above will fund and/or expand the curriculum?

including changes to clinical practice or new curriculum. When a stakeholder's readiness for change is high, they are more likely to embrace innovation and demonstrate a higher commitment during the implementation process. This is especially critical when challenges during the implementation processes are encountered. In contrast, when readiness to change is low, resistance to adopt the innovation prevails, complicating the implementation process and potentially leading to innovation adoption failure. The relationship between evidence-based medical innovations and clinical practice depicts these scenarios.[21] Although medicine is rich with generating scientific discoveries, implementing these innovations within clinical practice and across an entire health care delivery system is often reported as unreliable, variable, and difficult to scale because of a failure in recognizing the different states of readiness across and within an organization. Hence, diagnosing the readiness for change in key stakeholders is a critical step.

Diagnosing a stakeholder's readiness within an institution can draw from the seminal work from Everett Rogers. His diffusion of innovation model categorizes adopters of innovation into five groups: innovators (the fastest adopters with a high tolerance for risk), early adopters (often leadership who create legitimacy and accelerate the innovation), the early and late majority (view change more localized and generally risk averse, with the late majority hinging decisions based on the early majority), and laggards (traditionalists with rational reasons to resist change).[22] Fig. 1.3 describes the distribution of categories of adopters of innovation likely found across members within an institution.

For example, an assistant dean who might be an innovator of HSS at their institution must consider the readiness for change of the chair of the academic department responsible for the learning environment adopting HSS during the engagement process. If the chair is an early adopter, their

likelihood for change will rely on the assistant dean to communicate the generalizability of HSS that meets an array of factors across an institution, including how HSS would be socialized for institutional legitimacy purposes. Furthermore, if the chair is categorized as a laggard, they may be easily misconstrued as an obstructionist. The assistant dean should consider the chair's perspective, including their incentives with allocating scarce resources and time and correspondingly propose how to mitigate those constraints. Completing the templates in Tables 1.1 and 1.2 will identify key workgroup partners to mitigate constraints and catalyze the process of forming a high-reliability team.

Stakeholder recognition and engagement is a critical step to building consensus and a shared vision in implementing an HSS curriculum. As key stakeholders are identified and sorted into different phases of the implementation process, forming and mobilizing those who will be part of the day-to-day operations team is the next step.

Develop a Shared Vision and Strategy

Developing a shared vision and strategy among these newly identified stakeholders facilitates an institution's readiness to implement an HSS curriculum. This shared vision and strategy also must concurrently consider shared outcomes. Readiness for change, the value that will be added to the current state and existing assets through HSS integration, links to the overarching institutional mission, and the best ways to approach barriers are critical issues that must be fully considered before proceeding to implementation.

The concept of co-production recognizes diverse perspectives in creating a shared vision and strategy. Co-production identifies shared outcomes across stakeholders and is reported to promote alignment of outcomes and dismantle silos across health professionals training. Additionally, it incorporates the systemness, aligning the health care delivery systems with health professionals training to foster the vision of a "learning health system" across competing goals within academic health centers.[23,24] Incorporating co-production into the pre-implementation planning allows for "knowledge, vision, values, and cultures to be mutually developed between stakeholders" to identify shared assets and crystallize shared outcomes.[24]

During the pre-implementation planning process, an HSS curricular design team in the education space working with stakeholders in the delivery system could incorporate co-production by identifying their commonalities. For example, quality improvement is now a commonly expected component in the health care delivery system to facilitate continuous improvement of care, as observed in UME with the AAMC's QIPS and required of the GME learning environment.[9,25] Co-producing an HSS curriculum centered on patient safety and systems thinking in conjunction with

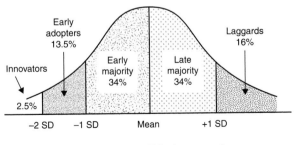

Fig. 1.3 Categories of innovation adoption. *SD,* Standard deviation. (Data from Rogers E. *Diffusion of Innovations.* 5th ed. Free Press; New York, NY; 2003.)

an existing quality improvement project offers an opportunity for stakeholders to convene and recognize their shared needs and assets and plan shared outcomes that meet each respective stakeholder's goals. This step aligns stakeholders in a shared vision with a sense of urgency that provides the requisite momentum to the rest of the HSS curriculum integration process.

Next, we will discuss the importance of building highly effective teams, including why it is necessary, what an ideal team looks like, how to attract the right team members, how to ensure they work well together, how to apply HSS domains to team activities, and how to maximize team effectiveness.

BUILDING HIGHLY EFFECTIVE TEAMS FOR HEALTH SYSTEMS SCIENCE IMPLEMENTATION

As with any broad educational endeavor, the successful and sustainable integration of HSS curricula and initiatives relies in great part on the formation of a **high-reliability** team to drive these efforts. Whether in the process of organizational and stakeholder engagement or other aspects of pre-implementation planning, the value of highly effective teams is immeasurable. Such teams are typically distinguished by interwoven characteristics that underlie their operational effectiveness, organizational agility, and ability to effect change. Although there is no single model of team effectiveness that has universally emerged as superior, the common elements of each model can be distilled into accessible principles that have the potential to catalyze this work. Several models are worth noting for their demonstrated value in dynamic organizational environments. In this section, we consider the value of interprofessional and interdisciplinary teams and team science to the integration of HSS curriculum across systems. We also describe the characteristics that underlie the success of these teams and strategies to overcome the inherent challenges that even the most effective teams encounter in their work. In addition, Table 1.3 provides examples of how characteristics of effective teamwork can be considered in the context of HSS implementation.

Why Teamwork?

As described, the engagement of key stakeholders, albeit organizational leaders or collaborators in the clinical learning environment, is requisite to building the consensus required to advance the work of HSS across the learning continuum. After this consensus is achieved, the next phase prioritizes the creation of high-reliability, outcomes-driven teams to advance the work. Effective teamwork skills are an expected professional competency across nearly all industries and disciplines. Whether in the quest to provide outstanding patient care or to solve the challenges posed by modern medical education, it is apparent that the critical thinking, relational skills, and cross-sectional workflows that underlie teamwork traverse professions and disciplines.

What Does the Ideal Team Look Like?

The ideal team composition varies based on need and audience. An ideal HSS team would, at its core, include representation across most, if not all, sectors of the medical education learning continuum in addition to subject content expertise. The rationale for this reflects the need to consider HSS as "vernacular" of medicine, in which all members of the team, whether a medical student, clinical trainee, interprofessional colleague, or faculty member, are fluent. The impact of engaging medical students for example, in such "value-added roles" is well-described by Gonzalo et al.[7] Their characterization of the "guiding coalition," as described in Fig. 1.1, echoes the importance of including both early and advanced learners as HSS teams form. Thus, for a UME-directed HSS curriculum, medical students on a rotating basis would work alongside clerkship directors, course directors, curricular deans, interprofessional colleagues, health system leaders, and administrative team members to define learning objectives, plan and review assessments, and identify learning activities for HSS curriculum implementation. Although seemingly daunting, this planning aspect of HSS is an important adjunct to the experiential component to which students are exposed in the clinical learning environment. The real-world perspective that students bring to the process of HSS planning enables leaders to more effectively reflect the goals and competencies that today's learners will need for successful practice in the future.

Likewise, today's clinical trainees are facing unprecedented challenges and new expectations in a health system that has never before been so complex and dynamic. As with undergraduate HSS teams, those working within the GME space must prioritize the engagement of trainees to partner with designated institutional officers, program directors, quality and safety leaders, interprofessional team members, and even patients to maximize the frame of systems thinking that underlies HSS curriculum implementation. What optimal HSS teams will derive from the engagement of trainees is an understanding of the critical issues facing training physicians and the competency gaps that resident and fellow physicians may identify through self-reflection and formal assessments. This information can be applied to guide curriculum development and refinement. Similarly, the inclusion of patients in select stages of HSS implementation can target assessment of competency attainment through such methods as 360 evaluations.

TABLE 1.3 Crosswalk Between Characteristics of Effective Teamwork and Health Systems Science Implementation

Characteristic of Effective Teamwork	Description	Key Considerations in Health Systems Science (HSS) Implementation	Examples
Conditions	• Most essential characteristic for effective team performance • Requires understanding of the environment and readiness for change • Includes assessment of not only gaps in knowledge but also culture, readiness for change, and the available resources	• Conduct environmental scan or needs assessment during the pre-implementation phase of HSS implementation • Consider what aspects of organizational or institutional culture will either enable HSS to thrive or pose barriers to success • Engage with stakeholders to understand opportunities, concerns, and challenges to HSS implementation	• The curriculum dean for undergraduate medical education maps the curriculum against key HSS competencies to identify opportunities for enhancement • The assistant dean of graduate medical education conducts a gap analysis across affiliate hospitals to elicit common themes across the areas of health care quality and patient safety in the clinical learning environment
Capability	• Honestly evaluate how team member experiences and skills (capability) may advance the work of HSS integration • Foster a mindset that supports growth and innovation	• Prioritize diversity of experience and thought when engaging HSS implementation teams (e.g., inclusion of interprofessional colleagues, learners, and patients) • Recognize that contributions from those with experience from other realms similar to, but not identical to, HSS may accelerate progress • Do not assume that other educational leaders (e.g., course or program directors, deans, program staff) will possess the depth of expertise that HSS implementation teams do; be prepared to engage and educate to drive change	• The course director for the new health equity class that is required for all first-year medical students invites colleagues from the school of nursing and members of the hospital's family advisory council to join the opening panel for the course, titled "Why Should HSS Matter to You?" • The department chair provides support for faculty in their department to participate in a national mentoring program focused on HSS
Coordination	• Leverage a "collective efficacy," or coordination, to pivot and meet stakeholders where they are in the cycle of change management • Step back and appreciate the value of smaller gains in favor of far-reaching change	• Cultivate awareness of competing academic or system priorities and consider how these might impact goals of HSS implementation	• A core faculty member for HSS at the medical school has proposed a department-wide training for HSS that will be required for all faculty; the plan is met with resistance • The training is rescoped as optional for faculty, with continuing medical education (CME) credit offered to those who wish to participate

Continued

TABLE 1.3 Crosswalk Between Characteristics of Effective Teamwork and Health Systems Science Implementation—cont'd

Characteristic of Effective Teamwork	Description	Key Considerations in Health Systems Science (HSS) Implementation	Examples
Cognition	• Establish common goals, approach, and purpose • Confirm shared understanding and vision (cognition) • Emphasize areas of commonality and consensus	• When possible, remind individuals of the intersection between HSS and work they are already doing • Help individuals understand "why this matters to me" through alignment of goals and competencies, rather than specific learning activities • Lean on validated and established models of change management to facilitate strong connections between implementation teams and stakeholders	• During a GME committee meeting, the designated institutional officer presents an overview of the ACGME CLER Program and the intersection between the program focus areas and HSS • The medical school dean shares comparative data during a curriculum committee meeting, reflecting how HSS has been implemented at peer institutions
Communication	• High emotional intelligence and keen situational awareness provide the implicit cues to guide progress in the most effective teams • Consider the importance of communication within the team, although messaging to stakeholders is equally important	• Know the audience and tailor messaging to the respective level of interest and understanding of HSS • Acknowledge contributions and express appreciation often • Be prepared for challenges and resistance to implementation; react without reacting	• The feedback from an inaugural elective focused on HSS in the clinical learning environment is poor; the course director is trying to make the case for continued FTE support to lead the course • Collate experiences from broad data sources, including comparative peer data, to demonstrate the slow initial uptake of HSS across some institutions, with subsequent acceleration
Conflict	• Not readily avoidable • Must differentiate task from process or relational conflict • Can stimulate innovation or action	• By their nature, HSS imperatives may introduce conflict within organizations, health systems, and institutions, particularly because its implementation and associated metrics for success have not been standardized across the learning continuum	• At an executive leadership meeting, the medical school dean requests more budget support to fund core faculty teaching for HSS, among other educational initiatives • The COO points out recent overall losses in clinical productivity among faculty and thus their reluctance to allocate more funds to teaching • A working group is proposed by the school dean to establish targets for and to evaluate the correlation between time spent in educational activities versus clinical productivity of core HSS faculty members

TABLE 1.3 Crosswalk Between Characteristics of Effective Teamwork and Health Systems Science Implementation—cont'd

Characteristic of Effective Teamwork	Description	Key Considerations in Health Systems Science (HSS) Implementation	Examples
Coaching	• Effective leadership (coaching) supports both the team and task • Coaching may be required for content and change management to achieve success	• Lead through the frame of encouragement, support, and empowerment for collaborators in HSS implementation	• The attending receives a cumulative report of their clinical teaching during their annual faculty evaluation; they are noted by trainees to spend "too much time on things that don't really matter on a day-to-day basis," namely nonclinical topics such as health care economics, ethics, and clinical informatics • The division chief offers feedback and encourages the attending to continue teaching on these topics while making a more intentional and explicit connection between the experiences of their trainees in the clinical learning environment to these core HSS concepts
Cooperation	• "Collective orientation" (cooperation) enables teams to prioritize the good of the whole over individual desires • Reflects a team commitment to transparency and a willingness to accept feedback	• Acknowledge progress in implementation, even if the ultimate goal is not yet fully realized • Cultivate an environment for safe dialogue within the HSS team and with key stakeholders regarding opportunities for improvement	• An organization-wide module is launched to train all medical staff in HSS. The training focuses on several key elements of HSS; however, it has been significantly scaled back from its initial version to shorten the duration of the training module • The authors of the module create a revised timeline to represent a phased approach and scale-up for training in HSS among all medical staff, including incentives for early adoption

ACGME, Accreditation Council for Graduate Medical Education; *CLER,* Clinical Learning Environment Review; *COO,* chief operating officer; *FTE,* full-time equivalent; *GME,* graduate medical education.

How Do We Attract the Right Team Members?

Partners, advocates, and collaborators for HSS implementation vary from educators, clinicians, learners, and other workforce members. The construction of the team depends on the willful, active, and authentic participation of all individuals regardless of their background and experience. One challenge that may be more frequently encountered in HSS team composition is the heterogeneity of knowledge and experience that team members may bring regarding HSS. Although individuals may possess experience in specific domains of HSS, historically these areas of content expertise may not have been identified under the specific frame of HSS. This situation may result in missed opportunities to leverage the expertise of team members without intentional assessment of content knowledge. Additionally, although the construct of HSS has been relatively recently defined and formalized, it is still important to note the value of contributions for those colleagues who may have long been engaged in this work if only through a different framework.

Attracting the right team members to engage in HSS implementation requires establishment of a sense of urgency but also a clear understanding by stakeholders of how their participation directly benefits their own professional or personal goals.[7] Health system leaders, for example, may consider how the creation of incentive-based goals focused on HSS may catalyze their existent organizational work in areas such as value-based care, health equity, and population health. Similarly, educators may be driven by their responsibility to ensure that their learners acquire necessary competencies in HSS but equally motivated by the potential to engage in related scholarly activity that may be an output of HSS curricular implementation. Patients and populations that are at the center of why HSS is needed also derive value from engaging in the conversation, both through sharing the perspectives as the functional "end users" for the competencies that physicians and other health care professionals apply in their clinical practice.

How Do Teams Work Best Among Themselves and With Others?

Whether working internally or connecting with stakeholders, effective HSS curriculum implementation teams will not achieve excellence through complacency. Actionable steps, including team coaching and training, iterative assessment of team performance, and the establishment of an environment that supports **psychological safety** and humility, enable even strong teams to exceed their own best potential. Although seemingly implicit, the behaviors and attitudes that are exemplified by the most effective teams are amplified through team coaching and training. This is true whether for primarily knowledge or task-driven teams or mixed purpose teams, such as those for HSS implementation. Team coaching and training provides a space in which HSS teams that may be navigating complex and matrixed organizational structures and resistance to change or barriers to consensus can have open dialogue, plan strategically, and problem solve with the application of validated team training principles.[26] Similarly, teams that routinely assess and reassess their strengths, opportunities, and strategies are more likely to identify gaps early in the process and intervene as needed.

A culture of continuous quality improvement not only benefits the team but also the process.

What Is the Intersection Between Systems Thinking, Team Science, and Health Systems Science?

Whether in the clinical, basic, social, or translational sciences, the "collaborative efforts to address challenges through leveraging of the strengths and expertise of professionals trained in different fields," also known as **team science**, accelerates change, innovation, and achievement.[27] Across the learning continuum of medical education, such interprofessional team collaboration has been identified as an essential competency for professional practice.[28] Both in HSS and team science, the essential domains—teaming, leadership, communication, and change management—are organized around the needs of patient, family, and community, surrounded by a framework of interdependent and shared learning. A commitment to the key principles of team science (collaboration) and systems thinking (synthesis) enables teams to best leverage the essential domains of HSS—teaming, leadership, ethics, and change management—toward success in HSS implementation.

For each specific organization, the actualization of HSS implementation teams may vary; however, certain team member roles are commonly requisite for success. Table 1.4 describes the core functions that HSS implementation teams will need and associated positions typically found across the continuum of medical education that would perform these functions.

Strategies to Maximize Team Effectiveness

Even when the team characteristics are used during HSS implementation, the most effective teams continue to integrate additional tools and strategies into their workflows to promote sustained excellence and longitudinal quality improvement.[29-31] The application of team charters, checklists, structured debriefing tools, and standardized guidelines for the provision of feedback enhance the likelihood of success for HSS curricular teams. When used consistently, these resources create space for engagement and dialogue, promote shared understanding, and normalize the process of iterative review that is intrinsic to any new curriculum intervention or change. Synergistically and systematically, effective HSS curricular teams can navigate complex academic medical and clinical environments to facilitate competency and mastery acquisition in HSS across the learning continuum. After the team is formed, it can move forward with the initial steps to plan implementation, which include completing a needs assessment.

TABLE 1.4   Health Systems Science Core Team Examples

Core Health Systems Science (HSS) Implementation Team Function(s)	Key Skills or Capabilities Required to Execute Core Functions	Proposed Stakeholder or Individual to Perform Key Functions
• Develop and establish vision for HSS implementation within the organization or unit • Establish common goals, approach, and purpose to HSS implementation • Train faculty and other key stakeholders regarding the value of HSS implementation • Facilitate forums for engagement and feedback • Promote psychological safety	• Content expertise • Vision and passion for HSS • Organizational acumen and agility • Growth and innovation mindset • High emotional intelligence and keen situational awareness • Leadership experience or training • Commitment to collaboration, dialogue, and action	• Educational leader (dean; associate or assistant dean) • Designated institutional officer • Faculty member (significant experience with HSS)
• Create a project plan and timeline • Monitor and track team progress toward goals and deadlines • Facilitate communication, meetings, and collaboration between stakeholders	• Project management training or expertise • Experience with program development • Content knowledge • Attentiveness to detail and organizational skills • Process-driven and outcomes-focused attitude	• Project manager • Program or unit administrator
• Provide sponsorship for the vision for HSS implementation • Engage executive leaders • Advocate for sustainability • Enable resource allocation to support HSS implementation	• Understanding of organizational culture • Knowledge of key unit or organizational priorities and vision • Some content knowledge regarding HSS • Charisma, confidence, and trust • Willingness to challenge status quo • Ability to navigate conflict	• Executive leadership • Academic department chair
• Champion engagement and dissemination of HSS curricula across the unit or organization • Coach colleagues through successful HSS curriculum implementation	• Commitment to building and fostering collaborative relationships • Energy, enthusiasm, and tenacity	• Faculty member • Course director • Trainees • Students
• Evaluate and assess data from HSS implementation initiatives to guide continuous quality improvement • Develop tools or rubrics to enable analysis of the effectiveness of HSS outcomes • Collate experiences from broad data sources, including comparative peer data, to demonstrate the organizational impact of HSS implementation	• Assessment or evaluation methodologic training • Detail oriented • Content knowledge • Data visualization expertise	• PhD or EdD methodologist • Statistician or analyst • Faculty member

Continued

TABLE 1.4 Health Systems Science Core Team Examples—cont'd		
Core Health Systems Science (HSS) Implementation Team Function(s)	**Key Skills or Capabilities Required to Execute Core Functions**	**Proposed Stakeholder or Individual to Perform Key Functions**
• Partner with HSS implementation teams to disseminate the curriculum • Role model desired HSS knowledge, skills, and behaviors for learners • Embrace and catalyze change	• Content knowledge • Openness to change • Resourceful and innovative approach to teaching and learning	• Faculty • Trainees • Students • Leaders
• Support the integration of HSS curriculum in the learning environment • Raise opportunities for the application of HSS curriculum across different populations, including interprofessional colleagues and patients • Encourage permissive spaces for reflection, innovation, and dialogue	• Some content knowledge • Ability to communicate and advocate for specific needs related to the intersection of HSS curriculum implementation and the unique perspectives of the constituents they represent • Willingness to engage in collaborative learning models	• Interprofessional partners and colleagues • Patients and families • Other administrative units or teams (e.g., community groups, national organizations)

EVALUATING THE CURRENT STATE: EDUCATOR COMPETENCY, CURRICULAR STRUCTURE, AND THE LEARNING ENVIRONMENT

After a decision has been made to implement HSS curriculum at a given institution and recognition of its core domains and the key initial steps in pre-implementation are determined, the work of identifying existing assets begins. Educators with knowledge covering HSS core domains may be in place; however, faculty development or recruitment of content experts could be necessary to address gaps. The curricular structure (existing or planned) may or may not facilitate HSS topic integration. The learning environment supporting the entirety of biomedical, clinical, and existing HSS education may contain extensive curricular mappings to HSS domains, or it may be revealed that key concepts are lacking. These gaps in both curricular structures and learning environments provide areas of focus for HSS curriculum design and implementation.

Educator Competency

In established medical schools, there is likely significant expertise in HSS content domains, but educators may be unfamiliar with the term, its definition, and its breadth. A survey that identifies colleagues with existing interest or content expertise in HSS topics is essential because it can propel pre-implementation forward. This effort should include "nontraditional educators," extending to individuals in the legal, policy, public health, and other social science disciplines.[32] However, such a survey will likely identify opportunities that require focused faculty development as a component of pre-implementation.

It also is important to appreciate that even the most robust HSS content expertise does not spontaneously create educational excellence. Leveraging such an asset to inform appropriate curriculum design and pedagogies (including small group case discussions and simulations) comprises a critical step in HSS curriculum implementation.

Curricular Structure

At the UME level, an HSS curriculum before implementation will differ based on the structure (existing or planned) of the medical school curriculum as the process of change begins. A new institution planning its curriculum can potentially place HSS within the foundation of its curriculum design. In comparison, a program with an established curriculum and years away from major revision will have different, but similarly challenging, work ahead of it. However, a set of questions would apply to these and "in-between" settings and merit consideration as pre-implementation begins:

- Do established, program-wide competencies for UME adequately encompass the HSS content that will be integrated? If not, how and when will this be developed?

- Is HSS to be considered as distinct courses or blocks separated from other curricular elements? Will HSS be integrated more broadly across multiple courses?
- If the latter, will HSS content be positioned longitudinally from matriculation to graduation or only within certain curricular phases?
- Will a full range of HSS core domains be taught? Or are factors such as local expertise, available space within the curriculum, and institutional culture and mission expected to narrow the focus?

As discussed in Chapter 5, conceptualizing HSS curriculum development at the GME level presents a different set of challenges than UME. In the contexts of GME program requirements and core competencies, ACGME sets the expectations related to HSS core domains, including health system improvement, patient safety, health care inequities, systems-based practice, and evidence-based medicine.[10] Additionally, structurally, GME training is primarily designed for immersion in the clinical environment. Hence, only a subset of these questions may be relevant.

The Learning Environment

A key pre-implementation step is to study the existing learning environment, which includes but should extend beyond, understanding how an institution is addressing HSS alongside delivery of traditional biomedical and clinical curricular content. When considering HSS, focus should be on how the learning environment (including classroom, simulation, clerkships, and other learning settings) can help students develop knowledge, skills, and attitudinal behaviors that reflect the importance of the third pillar.

Evaluation of the learning environment is likely to benefit from a gap analysis designed to comprehensively review all curricular phases. Although this analysis will find that most modern medical education curricula include substantive HSS-related content, faculty may be unaware that they are teaching HSS. Similarly, learners may not recognize it or are hesitant to embrace HSS comparison with the status quo biomedical and clinical curriculum.[33]

Performing a keyword search in settings that leverage existing curriculum management software (e.g., OASIS or New Innovations[34,35]) can be an effective first step in mapping the presence of HSS content (as well as faculty with interest and expertise, as referenced previously). However, the search query must be disciplined to prevent "signal-to-noise ratio" issues. The appearance of HSS-related keywords does not imply the material is being effectively taught. Limiting a search to the names of HSS core domains as described by Fig. 1.2 is likely to be too narrow, but basing it on the entire glossary of an HSS textbook or similar reference will likely be too broad. A more balanced approach could start with a finite number of keywords connecting to an HSS core domain. For example, when considering structural and social determinants of health, including keywords such as *gender, race, ethnicity, built environment, health literacy,* and *education* helps inform the needs assessment while not overwhelming the search with material less likely to support the query.

Upon completion of this step, HSS content verification follows and is optimally based on the study of course content or learning objectives. This evaluation can be accomplished either by accessing it as a course review or discussion with the faculty teaching it. This step is likely to refine the search down to a finite number of "hits," showing existing HSS material within a functioning curriculum and facilitating a more in-depth investigation of HSS content.

As with current state needs assessments of faculty knowledge and curricular structure, analysis of the learning environment will also identify strengths and potential opportunities. Developing a worksheet (Table 1.5) to record the inventory of HSS core domain content can be helpful. This will inform an overall current state analysis.

Table 1.5 is an example inventory of HSS core domains (columns) by year of medical school training (rows). When it is complete, evaluation of existing assets will inform the next step in pre-implementation and potential engagement of additional team members, which may bring further context to the current needs assessment state.

TABLE 1.5 Current State Inventory of HSS Core Domain Content Template									
	Quality or Safety	Value	Structures or Processes	Population Health	Informatics	Policy or Economics	Teaming	Legal or Ethics	Systems Thinking
Year 1									
Year 2									
Year 3									
Year 4									
Electives									

COMPLETING THE PRE-IMPLEMENTATION PROCESS

As a planning team completes steps 1 to 4 of the change management process, proceeding with the full implementation process, as described in Fig. 1.1's steps 5 to 8, requires the team to identify shared goals that are specific, measurable, achievable, relevant, and time-based (SMART) and align with the stakeholder engagement process.[36] As specific curricular transformation efforts commence, incorporating the team's SMART goal as a guiding North Star will illuminate the steps to full implementation with trackable project milestone achievements. Through these data-driven steps, steps 5 to 8 are actualized and incorporated into the iterative process to scale and sustain the curriculum transformation process.

CONCLUSION

Pre-implementation is a foundational step upon which the implementation of HSS curriculum is built. The implementation journey requires an in-depth understanding of the HSS core functional domains, core foundational domains, and the linking domain in tandem with the principles of change management. Implementation should proceed only after a robust, current state assessment of HSS-related faculty knowledge and curricular characteristics. Ultimately, implementation success hinges upon engaging a broad range of stakeholders and creating effective teams that share a vision of holistic medical education and prominent inclusion of HSS. The following chapters continue the implementation journey, with Chapter 2 focusing on the HSS competencies.

TAKE-HOME POINTS

1. Pre-implementation is a vital prerequisite stage that antecedes implementation and predicts its successful pull through.
2. This stage also involves mapping the current state and conducting a needs assessment for curricular transformation.
3. Change management is a core component to curriculum development.
4. Pre-implementation includes gauging stakeholder readiness and state of change followed by stakeholder identification and the appreciation of the attributes of highly effective teams.
5. Before exiting the pre-implementation phase, there must be an approach to defining success and road-mapping the journey to ensure that the implementation of HSS curriculum can be tracked for milestone achievement and stakeholder enrollment with attainment of full implementation.

QUESTIONS FOR FURTHER THOUGHT

1. Is the institution ready to consider the changes necessary for HSS curriculum integration?
2. If so, which component in the medical education continuum (undergraduate medical education, graduate medical education, continuing medical education) is under consideration?
3. What assets and resources within the institution could facilitate HSS curriculum integration?
4. What barriers could be anticipated, and how will they be addressed?
5. Who should make up the team(s) that will sponsor, plan, and implement the HSS curriculum?

VIGNETTE

Jesse is an assistant dean of medical education overseeing the integration of HSS into their institution's existing curriculum, with plans to refresh the preclerkship cardiology cases for their MD program. Jesse needs to refresh and implement a case in the cardiology block taught over 12 hours per week for 6 weeks in conjunction with a weekly preceptorship in the clinical setting for 180 students over 3 campuses. To start, the congestive heart failure case is to address hospital readmissions, interprofessional collaborative teams, and the social and structural determinants of health.

In tandem, Jesse has also been asked by their dean to work with their institution's designated institutional officer (DIO), who oversees the Clinical Learning Environment Review (CLER) Program at their affiliated health system, which sponsors 28 Accreditation Councils for Graduate Medical Education–accredited residency programs across 10 specialties. In preparing for their next CLER visit, the DIO aims to implement quality improvement (QI) projects across a selection of residency programs and plans to incorporate HSS curriculum for residents and their QI projects to help close patient care gaps.

Thought Questions

1. What does Jesse need to get started?
2. What does Jesse need to be successful in both scenarios?
3. What are the assets that Jesse can build from?
4. What challenges will Jesse need to overcome?
5. How can Jesse adapt the principles of change management for their specific learning environment?

ANNOTATED BIBLIOGRAPHY

Berwick DM. Disseminating innovations in health care. *JAMA.* 2003;289(15):1969.

This article discusses the relationship between medical innovations and their adoption in the clinical practice setting using the diffusions of innovation model to explain how to incorporate and spread innovations for sustainable change. The author outlines three factors that influence the rate of diffusion for innovations: how the innovation is perceived, the characteristics of recipients to the innovation, and the contextual organizational and social factors that can support or resist the concept of change.

Buljac-Samardzic M, Doekhie KD, van Wijngaarden JDH. Interventions to improve team effectiveness within health care: a systematic review of the past decade. *Hum Resour Health.* 2020;18(1):2.

This systematic review examines the team science research that studied improving team functioning in the health care setting. Four intervention types and their effectiveness are discussed, including training programs, practice improvement tools, organizational redesign, and comprehensive programs that include teaming interventions.

Gonzalo JD, Chang A, Dekhtyar M, Starr SR, Holmboe E, Wolpaw DR. Health systems science in medical education: unifying the components to catalyze transformation. *Acad Med.* 2020; 95(9):1362-1372.

This article discusses how the third pillar of medical education, health systems science (HSS), provides a conceptual framework to align medical education with the clinical environment. It includes the guidance and rationale to crosswalk HSS topics with national systems-related competencies. The authors discuss how operationalizing systems-related competencies help develop systems citizens who can meet and transform the demands of the learning environment embedded in complex health care delivery systems.

Gonzalo JD, Lucey C, Wolpaw T, Chang A. Value-added clinical systems learning roles for medical students that transform education and health: a guide for building partnerships between medical schools and health systems. *Acad Med.* 2017; 92(5):602-607.

The authors across multiple institutions provide an integrated curriculum development framework for HSS to foster partnerships between the education and clinical settings, and to foster value-added roles for medical students. By integrating the Kotter change management model with the Kern curriculum development model, the authors outline a roadmap, complete with a stepwise process, to promote a synergistic relationship between medical education and the delivery system, and create a collaborative and optimal learning environment for medical students.

REFERENCES

1. Kotter JP. Leading change: why transformation efforts fail. *Harv Bus Rev.* May 1, 1995. <https://hbr.org/1995/05/leading-change-why-transformation-efforts-fail-2>; 1995 Accessed 08.04.22.
2. American Association of Medical Colleges. *Curriculum Change in U.S. Medical Schools.* AAMC. <https://www.aamc.org/data-reports/curriculum-reports/interactive-data/curriculum-change-medical-schools>; Accessed 25.06.22.
3. Skochelak SE, Hammond MM, Lomis KD, et al., eds. *Health Systems Science.* 2nd ed. St. Louis: Elsevier; 2020.
4. Gonzalo JD, Lucey C, Wolpaw T, Chang A. Value-added clinical systems learning roles for medical students that transform education and health: a guide for building partnerships between medical schools and health systems. *Acad Med.* 2017;92(5):602.
5. Gonzalo JD, Singh MK. *Building Systems Citizenship in Health Professions Education: The Continued Call for Health Systems Science Curricula.* Agency for Healthcare Research and Quality: Patient Safety Network. <https://psnet.ahrq.gov/perspective/building-systems-citizenship-health-professions-education-continued-call-health-systems>; 2019 Accessed 08.04.22.
6. Gonzalo JD, Dekhtyar M, Starr SR, et al. Health systems science curricula in undergraduate medical education: identifying and defining a potential curricular framework. *Acad Med.* 2017;92(1):123-131.
7. Gonzalo J, Hammoud MM, Schneider GW. *Value-Added Roles for Medical Students.* St. Louis: Elsevier; 2021.
8. Schuster MA, Conwell WD, Connelly MT, Humphrey HJ. Building equity, inclusion, and diversity into the fabric of a new medical school: early experiences of the Kaiser Permanente Bernard J. Tyson School of Medicine. *Acad Med.* 2020;95(suppl 2):S66.
9. American Association of Medical Colleges. *Quality Improvement and Patient Safety Competencies Across the Learning Continuum.* American Association of Medical Colleges; Rockville, MD; 2019.
10. Accreditation Council for Graduate Medical Education. *CLER Pathways to Excellence: Expectations for an Optimal Clinical Learning Environment to Achieve Safe and High-Quality Patient Care, Version 2.0.* Accreditation Council for Graduate Medical Education; Chicago, IL; 2019.

11. Edgar L, Roberts S, Holmboe E. Milestones 2.0: a step forward. *J Grad Med Educ.* 2018;10(3):367-369.

12. Nelson EC, Batalden PB, Huber TP, et al. Microsystems in health care: part 1. Learning from high-performing front-line clinical units. *Jt Comm J Qual Improv.* 2002;28(9):472-493.

13. World Bank. *Mortality Rate, Infant (Per 1,000 Live Births), United States.* <https://data.worldbank.org/indicator/SP.DYN.IMRT.IN?locations=US>; Accessed 25.06.22

14. Commonwealth Fund. *U.S. Health Care From a Global Perspective, 2019: Higher Spending, Worse Outcomes?* <https://www.commonwealthfund.org/publications/issue-briefs/2020/jan/us-health-care-global-perspective-2019>; 2020 Accessed 07.06.22.

15. Martin AB, Hartman M, Lassman D, Catlin A, The National Health Expenditure Accounts Team. National health care spending in 2019: steady growth for the fourth consecutive year: study examines national health care spending for 2019. *Health Aff (Millwood).* 2021;40(1):14-24.

16. Bureau UC. *Health Insurance Coverage in the United States: 2020.* Census.gov. <https://www.census.gov/library/publications/2021/demo/p60-274.html>; 2021 Accessed 08.04.22.

17. Panagioti M, Khan K, Keers RN, et al. Prevalence, severity, and nature of preventable patient harm across medical care settings: systematic review and meta-analysis. *BMJ.* 2019;366:l4185.

18. Medscape. *Medscape National Physician Burnout & Suicide Report 2020: The Generational Divide.* Medscape. <https://www.medscape.com/slideshow/2020-lifestyle-burnout-6012460>; Accessed 25.06.22.

19. Gonzalo JD, Chang A, Dekhtyar M, Starr SR, Holmboe E, Wolpaw DR. Health systems science in medical education: unifying the components to catalyze transformation. *Acad Med.* 2020;95(9):1362-1372.

20. Centers for Disease Control and Prevention. *Program Evaluation Guide, Step 1.* <https://www.cdc.gov/evaluation/steps/step1/index.htm. >; 2020 Accessed 25.06.22.

21. Berwick DM. Disseminating innovations in health care. *JAMA.* 2003;289(15):1969.

22. Rogers E. *Diffusion of Innovations.* Free Press; 5th ed. New York, NY; 2003.

23. Holmboe ES, Batalden P. Achieving the desired transformation: thoughts on next steps for outcomes-based medical education. *Acad Med.* 2015;90(9):1215-1223.

24. Gonzalo JD, Dekhtyar M, Caverzagie KJ, et al. The triple helix of clinical, research, and education missions in academic health centers: a qualitative study of diverse stakeholder perspectives. *Learn Health Syst.* 2020;5(4):e10250.

25. Accreditation Council for Graduate Medical Education. *ACGME Common Program Requirements (Residency).* July 1, 2020. https://www.acgme.org/globalassets/PFAssets/ProgramRequirements/CPRResidency2020.pdf. Accessed June 25, 2022.

26. Lacerenza CN, Marlow SL, Tannenbaum SI, Salas E. Team development interventions: evidence-based approaches for improving teamwork. *Am Psychol.* 2018;73(4):517-531.

27. Steer CJ, Jackson PR, Hornbeak H, McKay CK, Sriramarao P, Murtaugh MP. Team science and the physician-scientist in the age of grand health challenges: team science and the physician-scientist. *Ann NY Acad Sci.* 2017;1404(1):3-16.

28. Lomis K, Amiel JM, Ryan MS, et al. Implementing an entrustable professional activities framework in undergraduate medical education: early lessons from the AAMC Core Entrustable Professional Activities for Entering Residency Pilot. *Acad Med.* 2017;92(6):765.

29. Buljac-Samardzic M, Doekhie KD, van Wijngaarden JDH. Interventions to improve team effectiveness within health care: a systematic review of the past decade. *Hum Resour Health.* 2020;18(1):2.

30. Lemieux-Charles L, McGuire WL. What do we know about health care team effectiveness? A review of the literature. *Med Care Res Rev.* 2006;63(3):263-300.

31. Hackman JR. Learning more by crossing levels: evidence from airplanes, hospitals, and orchestras. *J Org Behav.* 2003;24(8):905-922.

32. Gonzalo JD, Chang A, Wolpaw DR. New educator roles for health systems science: implications of new physician competencies for U.S. medical school faculty. *Acad Med.* 2019;94(4):501-506.

33. Gonzalo JD, Ogrinc G. Health systems science: the "broccoli" of undergraduate medical education. *Acad Med.* 2019;94(10):1425-1432.

34. Schilling Consulting. *OASIS Scheduling Software.* <http://www.schillingconsulting.com/oasis_scheduling.html>; Accessed 25.06.22.

35. New Innovations. *New Innovations—UME.* <https://www.new-innov.com/pub/ume.html>; Accessed 25.06.22.

36. Doran GT. There's a S.M.A.R.T. way to write management's goals and objectives. *Manage Rev.* 1981;70(11):35-36.

Health Systems Science Competencies in Medical Education

Jed Gonzalo, Sally A. Santen, Kimberly D. Lomis, and Maya M. Hammoud

LEARNING OBJECTIVES

1. List health systems science (HSS) core competencies.
2. Describe the relationship between HSS competencies and existing accreditation standards.
3. Apply HSS competencies in undergraduate, graduate, and interprofessional education.

CHAPTER OUTLINE

Chapter Summary, 19
Introduction, 19
   Health Systems Science Intersection with Medical Education Accreditation and National Curricula, 20
   Systems-Based Practice and Health Systems Science, 20

Competencies in Health Systems Science, 20
Health Systems Science Competencies Across the Continuum, 21
Discussion, 21
Take-Home Points, 31
Questions for Further Thought, 31

CHAPTER SUMMARY

Medical schools, residency programs, faculty development, and continuing medical education (CME) programs are seeking to optimally align educational experiences with the needs of patients, health systems, and society. Therefore, there is a pressing need to educate students and residents to become "systems ready" with a specific set of health systems science (HSS) skills and competencies upon their graduation. The HSS framework provides a comprehensive model for educators and learners to integrate into learning and care delivery.

This chapter describes the work of the American Medical Association (AMA) Accelerating Change in Medical Education Consortium's HSS competency workgroup. This group developed core competencies and associated key concepts in HSS that can be used as a foundation for acting upon recommendations in subsequent chapters of this book regarding curriculum design and implementation for undergraduate medical education (UME; preclerkship, clerkship, and postclerkship phases), graduate medical education (GME), and interprofessional collaboration.

INTRODUCTION

As health care undergoes significant transformation, medical schools along with residency, faculty development, and CME programs are seeking to optimally align educational experiences to the needs of health systems in the coming years. Notably, health systems leaders and educators have identified the pressing need to educate students to become "systems ready" upon their graduation from medical school, thereby rapidly acclimating in health systems where new skills are required.[1-3] A key area identified in UME to prepare students for changing practice environments is the enhancement of learning in HSS.[4] As described in Chapter 1, HSS is considered a third pillar of medical education that complements the basic and clinical sciences and includes concepts related to health care delivery, policy, clinical informatics, population and public health, value-based care, and health system improvement.[2,4]

Health systems science provides a comprehensive framework to improve patient and population care. The basic and clinical sciences reach their full potential through the full integration with HSS to ultimately impact patient health and achieve the **Quadruple Aim**—improving the patient experience of care, bettering the health of populations, reducing the per capita cost of health care, and increasing health care professional wellness.[5,6] The HSS framework cohesively unites previously scattered systems-related competencies and is now being used by many medical schools and residency programs. Because the foundations of HSS have a long history, there are many intersections of HSS across multiple domains. Many of these areas have articulated content, curricula, assessments, and competencies encompassed in HSS. This chapter discusses a few of these relationships and then describes the proposed competencies from the AMA Accelerating Change in Medical Education Consortium's HSS competency workgroup. Tables 2.1 and 2.2 illustrate the intersections of HSS with other frameworks and curricula.

Health Systems Science Intersection With Medical Education Accreditation and National Curricula

For medical students, HSS is incorporated in several areas.[38,39] The Liaison Committee on Medical Education (LCME) Standards and Data Collection Instrument, with supporting data from the Association of American Medical Colleges (AAMC) Graduation Questionnaire includes HSS topics. The content in the United States Medical Licensing Examination includes some areas of HSS as well. Additionally, the AAMC Core EPA for Entering Residency includes HSS topics.

Finally, there are several groups that have developed competencies related to HSS.[38] For quality improvement (QI) and patient safety (PS), the Institute of Medicine and the AAMC have focused on creating QI and PS curriculum and competencies across the continuum of medical education to provide a roadmap for curricular and professional development, assessment, and improvement of health care services and outcomes.[40] For interprofessional education and collaboration, aligned with the requirements of the LCME standards, nearly every medical school has implemented curricular areas in interprofessional education and collaboration. The Interprofessional Education Collaborative (IPEC) core competencies have identified four core competency domains: (1) values and ethics, (2) roles and responsibilities for collaborative practice, (3) interprofessional

communication, and (4) teamwork and team-based care.[41] These are described in more detail in Chapter 6. For the social determinants of health (SDH), influenced in part by the AAMC recommendation to increase SDH and behavioral health into curricula in 2007, medical education has seen an increase in education about factors related to health outcomes, such as food insecurity, social networks, and zip codes.[42] For high-value care, the American College of Physicians and Alliance for Academic Internal Medicine have defined the steps for implementing high-value care in clinical care settings and shared decision making.[43] Although each of these discrete areas is critical for learners across the continuum, each must be applied in a cohesive educational program to integrate in the mind and skill set of learners. The HSS framework provides a comprehensive model for educators and learners to integrate into learning and care delivery.

Systems-Based Practice and Health Systems Science

In 1999, the Accreditation Council for Graduate Medical Education (ACGME) established **systems-based practice** (SBP) as one of six core competencies in its vision of resident education.[44] The SBP competency articulated several underrepresented areas in medical education, all of which aimed to close the gap between patient and health system needs and the education of physicians.[45] The early iteration of SBP identified multiple HSS domains, such as interprofessional collaboration, high-value care, and understanding the larger context of health care environments.[46] More recently, the ACGME developed the harmonized milestones across all specialties recognizing the universal components of competency for physicians.[47] The opportunity of SBP, in part, lies in the ability of medical educators to operationalize a clear strategy that prioritizes and integrates HSS competencies with other competency areas and across the continuum.

COMPETENCIES IN HEALTH SYSTEMS SCIENCE

Despite the identification of curricular areas for HSS in medical education, there is an unmet need in identifying the competencies that should be expected at the student and intern levels. Building on the competency definition as "knowledge, skills, attitudes, and personal qualities essential to the practice of medicine" by Albanese et al (Box 2.1),[48] students and early residents need to be trained and assessed on HSS competencies.

This chapter builds on the work of the AMA Accelerating Change in Medical Education Consortium to propose core competencies in HSS. These core competencies and associated key concepts can be used as a foundation for acting on recommendations in subsequent chapters of this book regarding curriculum design and implementation for UME (pre-clerkship, clerkship, and postclerkship phases), GME, and interprofessional collaboration. Kern's six-step approach to curriculum development emphasizes backward design, in which the curriculum builds from objectives through implementation toward the goal of trainee competency in HSS.[49] Curriculum developers will need to integrate across core domains of HSS to align objectives, appropriate learning experiences, and rigorous assessments to ensure skill development in desired HSS competencies.

It is important to highlight one of the foundational competencies within this HSS framework—**systems thinking**.[50–53] The tools and strategies of systems thinking have emerged in the medical and public health education literature in past years. Systems thinking integrates the context of an individual's work in health care with a larger understanding of all components of the health system and a goal of working with these parts to achieve ideal outcomes. This concept is related to structural competency. In addition to specific skills and habits of work, systems thinking serves as a fundamental orientation to one's role. Being a physician is more than a skill set of diagnosing and providing a therapeutic plan for one patient. A new view of the systems thinker professionalism includes accountability to a community of physicians and other health care professionals working together to enhance the care of patients and populations.[53]

HEALTH SYSTEMS SCIENCE COMPETENCIES ACROSS THE CONTINUUM

Competency is a developmental process. However, in outlining the HSS competencies, we purposely avoided reference to specific levels of training. Because most physicians across the continuum have not received training in HSS, there is no expectation that competency aligns with level of training. Indeed, in many HSS domains, learners may be more advanced than practicing physicians. Unlike the development of clinical skills, in which the education community has rich experience to describe expected competency at various levels of training, the typical trajectory of development in HSS remains unknown and is an area of current research.[54] This chapter thus describes core competencies in HSS and provides a list of key representative concepts associated with each. Users of this text may refer to the Dreyfus model of expertise development to define expected levels of performance for their programs.[55–57] This model describes patterns of knowledge, interactions, and behaviors within the context of complex systems that

are associated with novice, advanced beginner, competent, proficient, and expert performance (Table 2.3). Educational designers must implement purposeful assessment tools to ascertain competency development aligned with programmatic goals. Collaboration within the education community is underway to develop assessment tools capable of distinguishing advanced competency in HSS.

Table 2.4 illustrates the final set of HSS competencies. These were developed through a several-phase approach. In the first phase, we asked each of the 32 AMA Accelerating Change in Medical Education Consortium member medical schools to submit any competencies that could potentially relate to HSS. One investigator was assigned each domain, and each conducted a literature review of existing learning objectives and competencies in medical education with preference for UME but not excluding other levels or disciplines (e.g., GME, CME, public health). These formed the early foundation of the work. The HSS competency workgroup then reviewed this material and consolidated it into the current framework. Last, the framework was refined and finalized by us, a subgroup of the initial HSS competency workgroup. The final framework is presented here as a living document because the core competencies are expected to endure, but nuances of training and performance, particularly at the proficient and expert levels, must change to correspond with changes in the health system and the evolving needs of patients and communities. Areas that are currently represented as key concepts, such as structural racism or artificial intelligence, may expand over time to generate more replete associated competencies. An outcomes-driven educational design is recommended so that programs can be responsive as competency needs evolve.

DISCUSSION

Competency in HSS is anticipated to support the Quadruple Aim: improving population health, enhancing patient experience, reducing health care costs, and improving health care professional wellness.[6] Many practicing physicians currently view themselves as victims of the health systems in which they work. Competency in HSS empowers physicians to improve these systems for the betterment of all stakeholders.

The HSS competencies are explicitly contextualized within the health care delivery system. A unique consideration regarding demonstration of competency is that these HSS competencies rely on one's interactions with other health care team members and with systems. Assessment tools that move beyond individual performance to that of the team or unit are required to realize the full potential of HSS. Given HSS curricula are in nascent stages, the

TABLE 2.1 Schema Crosswalk[a] of Health Systems Science (HSS) Learning Areas With Systems-Related National Competency Recommendations and Accreditation Standards

	HSS DOMAINS AND SUBDOMAINS																						
	PEC			HCD	PE		CIHT			PPH			HVC			QI		HSI					
Representative Examples	Pe	B	S	P	Po	EP	I	DS	T	SDH	Pu	PHI	Q	C	E	QI	D	IS	ST	CMA	EL	L	TW
UME Competency Recommendations and Accreditation Standards																							
AAMC Core EPAs for Entering Residency[7]	•			••					•	•			•	•	••	••							••
Competency domains for health professions[8]	•			•		•	•	•	•	•		•	•	•	•	•		•		•	•	•	••
Interprofessional education or collaborative care competencies[9]	•			••			•		•	•		•	•		•	•					•	•	••
IHI knowledge domains for improvement[10]	•	•	•	•		•		•	•									•	•		•	•	•
AAMC QI and PS competencies[11]	•		•	•		•	•	•	••	••		••	••	••	••	••	••				•		••
AAMC GQ (1998–2004)[b,c]	•		•	•	•	•	•	•	•	•	•		•	•	•					•	•		•
AAMC GQ (2005–2009)[b,c]	•		•	•	•	•	•	•		•	•		•	•	•	•				•	•		•
AAMC GQ (2010–2017)[b,c]	•		•	•		•	•	•	•	•	•	•	•		•	•					•	•	•
LCME Data Collection Instrument[12]	••		•	•		•	•	•	•		•	•	•								•		••
USMLE physician tasks and competencies[13]				•	•									•					•				
USMLE content outline[14]	•		•	•		•	•	•	•		•	•	••	•	••	••					•	•	••

GME Competency Recommendations and Accreditation Standards

ACGME SBP competency domain[15,16]		••	••			•		•	••	•	•		••
ACGME SBP, ICS, PBLI, and PRO milestones[17]	••	•	•	•	••	•	•	•	•	•	•	•	••
ACGME Common Program Requirements[18]		••				••		••	•	•			••
ACGME CLER Pathways to Excellence[19]		••	•	•	•	••		••	•	•	•		•

aSupplemental Digital Appendix 1 (http://links.lww.com/ACADMED/A906) describes methods used in performing the schema crosswalk; the • and •• designations were determined by investigators and represent degree of focus dedicated to an HSS area (i.e., • = minor focus, •• = moderate or high focus).

bSource: Association of American Medical Colleges Data Warehouse Codebooks, Graduation Questionnaire. Used with special permission.

cQuestions on the AAMC GQ only included items related to perceived preparedness for residency or to the time devoted to topics in curricula (and excluded binary items related to whether a concept or item was "used" in their experience).

AAMC, Association of American Medical Colleges; ACGME, Accreditation Council for Graduate Medical Education; CIHT, clinical informatics and health technology (DS, decision support; I, informatics; T, technology); CLER, Clinical Learning Environment Review; CMA, change management and advocacy; EL, ethics and legal; EPAs, entrustable professional activities; GME, graduate medical education; GQ, Graduation Questionnaire; HCD, health care delivery (S, structure; P, process); HSI, health system improvement (D, data and measurement; IS, innovation and scholarship; QI, quality improvement principles; HVC, high-value care (C, cost and waste; E, evaluation and metrics; Q, quality [including patient safety, effectiveness, efficiency, timeliness, patient-centered care, and equitable care]); ICS, interpersonal and communication skills; IHI, Institute for Healthcare Improvement; L, leadership; LCME, Liaison Committee on Medical Education; PBLI, practice-based learning and improvement; PE, policy and economics (EP, economics and payment; Po, policy); PEC, patient experience and context (B, behaviors and motivation; Pe, patient experience); PPH, population, public, and social determinants of health (PHI, population health and improvement; Pu, public health; SDH, social determinants of health); PRO, professionalism; PS, patient safety; SBP, systems-based practice; ST, systems thinking; TW, teamwork, teaming, and collaboration; UME, undergraduate medical education; USMLE, United States Medical Licensing Examination.

(Reprinted with permission from Gonzalo J, Chang A, Dekhtyar M, Starr S, Holmboe E, Wolpaw D. Health systems science in medical education: unifying the components to catalyze transformation. Acad Med. 2020;95:1362-1372.)

TABLE 2.2 Schema Crosswalk[a] of Health Systems Science (HSS) Learning Areas With Systems-Related National and Local Curricula, Educator Recommendations, and Textbooks

Representative Examples	HSS DOMAINS AND SUBDOMAINS																						
	PEC			HCD		PE		CIHT		PPH			HVC				HSI						
	Pe	B	S	Po	P	EP	I	DS	T	SDH	Pu	PHI	Q	C	E	QI	D	IS	ST	CMA	EL	L	TW
National and Local Curricula																							
IHI Open School curriculum[20]	••		•	•				•		••	•	•	••	••	•	••	••	••	•	••		••	••
ACP High Value-Care curriculum[21]	•			•		•							••	••	••	••	•	•					
Quality & Safety Educators Academy[22]			•	•									••		••	•	•			•		•	•
Harvard Medical School social medicine course[23]	•			•		•	•			••	••	•	•							•	•	•	•
Teachers of Quality Academy[24]			•	•			•	•		•	•	•	•	•	•	••	•	•	•	•			••
Mayo Clinic Alix SOM Science of HCD curriculum[25-27]	••	••	•	••		••	•	•	•	•	•	••	••	••	••	••	•	•	•	•	•	••	••
Educator Recommendations																							
UME Health Policy Curricula[28,29]	•		•	••		••	•	•	•	•	•	•	•	•	•	•					•	•	•
Clinical Prevention and Population Health Curriculum Framework[30]	•		•	••		•	•	•	•	••	••	••	•	•						•	•		
Population Health Curricular Framework[31]	•		•	•		•	•	•	•	•	•	••	•	•			•				•	•	•
UME-21 Initiative[32]			•	•				•		•	•	•	•	•									•

Textbooks

Population Health: Creating a Culture of Wellness[33]

Understanding Patient Safety[34]

Understanding Value-Based Healthcare[35]

Health Systems Science and Health Systems Science Review[36,37]

[a]Supplemental Digital Appendix 1 (http://links.1ww.com/ACADMED/A906) describes methods used in performing the schema crosswalk; the • and •• designations were determined by investigators and represent degree of focus dedicated to an HSS area (i.e., • = minor focus, •• = moderate or high focus). ACP, American College of Physicians; CIHT, clinical informatics and health technology (DS, decision support; I, informatics; T, technology); CMA, change management and advocacy; EL, ethics and legal; HCD, health care delivery (S, structure; P, process); HSI, health system improvement (D, data and measurement; IS, innovation and scholarship; QI, quality improvement principles); HVC, high-value care (C, cost and waste; E, evaluation and metrics; Q, quality [including patient safety, effectiveness, efficiency, timeliness, patient-centered care, and equitable care]); IHI, Institute for Healthcare Improvement; L, leadership; PE, policy and economics (EP, economics and payment; Po, policy); PEC, patient experience and context (B, behaviors and motivation; Pe, patient experience); PPH, population, public, and social determinants of health (PHI, population health and improvement; Pu, public health; SDH, social determinants of health); SOM, School of Medicine; ST, systems thinking; TW, teamwork, teaming, and collaboration; UME, undergraduate medical education.

(Reprinted with permission from Gonzalo J, Chang A, Dekhtyar M, Starr S, Holmboe E, Wolpaw D. Health systems science in medical education: unifying the components to catalyze transformation. Acad Med. 2020;95:1362-1372.)

BOX 2.1   Characteristics of a Competency

1. It should focus on the performance of the end product or goal-state of instruction.
2. It should reflect expectations that are an application of what is learned in the immediate instructional program.
3. It should be expressible in terms of measurable behavior; specifying the behaviors expected from competence is essential to being able to actually measure the attainment of the competency.
4. It should use a standard for judging competence that is not dependent upon the performance of other learners.
5. It should inform learners, as well as other stakeholders, about what is expected of them.

(Data from Albanese, Mark A, Mejicano G, Mullan P, Kokotailo P, Gruppen L. Defining characteristics of educational competencies. *Med Educ.* 2008;42(3):248-255.)

aspirational and expected ability of future physicians in a health care delivery model may not be totally realized as of yet. The process of creating these competencies was deliberately anticipatory of future needs, and the need for ongoing evolution of this work is acknowledged. This work may serve to catalyze alignment of health systems and health care delivery with the educational paradigm for learners across the continuum. The medical education community is continually seeking to educate physicians who will be health care "citizens," responsible members of health care teams, and stewards of health care resources. Defined competencies in HSS are an important framework to enculturate future physicians in communities of practice at the earliest point possible and foster continuing growth throughout one's career.

TABLE 2.3   Patterns of Knowledge, Interactions, and Behaviors Within the Context of Complex Systems That Are Associated With Novice, Advanced Beginner, Competent, Proficient, and Expert Performance

Stage	Characteristics
Novice	Rigid adherence to taught rules or plans Little situational perception No discretionary judgement
Advanced beginner	Guidelines for action based on attributes or aspects (aspects are global characteristics of situations recognizable only after some prior experience) Situational perception still limited All attributes and aspects are treated separately and given equal importance
Competent	Coping with crowdedness Now sees actions at least partially in terms of longer term goals Conscious, deliberate planning Standardized and routinized procedures
Proficient	Sees situations holistically rather than in terms of aspects Sees what is most important in a situation Perceives deviations from the normal pattern Decision-making less labored Uses maxims for guidance, whose meanings vary according to the situation
Expert	No longer relies on rules, guidelines, or maxims Intuitive grasp of situations based on deep tacit understanding Analytic approaches used only in novel situations or when problems occur Vision of what is possible

(Data from Dreyfus SE. *Four Models vs Human Situational Understanding: Inherent Limitations on the Modelling of Business Expertise,* ref F49620-79-C-0063. USAF Office of Scientific Research, 1981; Dreyfus HL, Dreyfus SE. Putting computers in their proper place: analysis versus intuition in the classroom. In: Sloan D, ed. *The Computer in Education: A Critical Perspective.* New York; Teachers' College Press; 1984 Wright-Patterson Air Force Base, Ohio.)

TABLE 2.4 Health Systems Science Competencies, Subcompetencies, and Key Concepts[a]

Core Domains, Subcompetencies, and Description	Key Representative Concepts
Domain 1: Systems Thinking	**Concepts related to the attention of a complex web of interdependence; an awareness of the "whole," not just the parts; and the ability to recognize multidirectional cause–effect relationships with all causes emerging as the effect of another system dynamics**
Systems thinking Applies knowledge, theory, techniques, and skills to enhance understanding of the interrelationships among elements, patterns of change, and structures underlying complex situations and health systems	Systems theory and systems dynamics Technical and complex adaptive systems Tools for analyzing interdependent systems (e.g., ladder of inference, iceberg, causal loops, connection circle) Habits demonstrated by systems thinkers (e.g., changes perspective to seek understanding, understands time delays) Structural competency
Domain 2: Health Care Delivery	**Concepts related to the organization of individuals, institutions, resources, and processes for delivery of health care to meet the needs of patients or populations of patients**
Structure of health care delivery Accounts for the structures of the health care system in the delivery and improvement of health care	Health care facilities and locations (e.g., nursing homes, long-term care facilities, operating rooms) Health care workforce (e.g., nurse practitioners, physicians, therapists) Resources available to address patient needs for preventive services, home health, and in postdischarge situations Features and principles of various health care delivery systems in US health care
Process of health care delivery Accounts for the processes of the health care system in the delivery and improvement of health care	Health care delivery; coordination of care; transitions of care, including discharging patients Intra- and interunit patient transfers Health information exchange Medication prescribing and reconciliation
Interprofessional collaborative care Collaborates with other health care professionals and coordinates care as required for optimal health care delivery (see IPCC competencies)	Values and ethics for interprofessional practice Roles and responsibilities of various health professionals Interprofessional communications Teams and teamwork
Domain 3: Policy and Economics	**Concepts related to the decisions, plans, and actions undertaken to achieve specific health care goals and the issues related to efficiency, effectiveness, value, and behavior in the production and consumption of health care. These sciences are used to promote health through the study of all components of the health care system and managed care**
Policy, law, and reform Recognizes and applies the impact of health care legislation on the US health care system, delivery of care, the practice of medicine, and the future of US health care	Various tiers of policy (e.g., national policy, e.g., Affordable Care Act, local policy, EMTALA); tort reform Triple and Quadruple Aims of health care delivery Analysis of current and future legislation to improve affordability and access to health care

Continued

TABLE 2.4   Health Systems Science Competencies, Subcompetencies, and Key Concepts[a]—cont'd

Core Domains, Subcompetencies, and Description	Key Representative Concepts
Economics and payment Appraises the consequences of health care economics and payment mechanisms on individual patient care, population health, and system performance and redesign	Fundamental components of health care coverage (e.g., Medicaid, Medicare, private insurance, exchanges) Health insurance concepts (e.g., co-pay, deductible); payment principles (e.g., capitation) Economic mechanisms (e.g., insurance markets, cost sharing) can affect costs, charges, and patient behavior Mechanisms for decreasing health care costs at the system level
Domain 4: Population and Public Health	**Concepts related to the full range of health determinants affecting entire populations (rather than just individuals), traditional public health, and preventive medicine, and the care and improvement in outcomes for populations of patients, specifically in regard to the dynamic interrelationships among various personal, socioeconomic, and environmental factors**
Social determinants of health Provides patient-centered care by assessing the conditions and factors impacting patient's ideal receipt of quality outcomes, inclusive of health-related features of neighborhoods, income, wealth, and education	Health care disparities and inequities The structural drivers of social determinants of health The impact of structural racism and other "-isms" on health The impact of context on health (including climate change)
Population health management Applies a synthetic, holistic approach to improving the patient health outcomes of a group of individuals, such as those from a specific geographic area or other characteristic	Theoretical models of rising risk (e.g., Kindig model); population measurement, assessment, and evaluation Populations: definitions (e.g., community, cohorts with disease states, populations of care, from panels to covered lives to health systems and accountable entities, geographic, political entities) Population management
Public health Recognizes importance of and integrates factors within communities, neighborhoods, and public health infrastructures to address patient and population health issues	Socioecological model Public health interventions Theory, definition, core functions, and essential services Relationship with medicine, health policy, and economics
Domain 5: Clinical Informatics and Technology	**Concepts related to the application of informatics and information technology to deliver health care services, including clinical decision support, documentation, electronic health records, and the utilization of data to improve health**
Health information technology Recognizes and integrates aspects of health care delivery related to technology systems that store, share, and analyze or share health information	Technology; EHR; health information exchange; telemedicine; confidentiality of data Professionalism in the application of data and information in the EHR Personal health records and patient portals to engage patients in improving health and care delivery Data sources to enact personalized medicine (e.g. -omic data, app data, patient reported outcomes, sensor data)

TABLE 2.4 Health Systems Science Competencies, Subcompetencies, and Key Concepts[a]—cont'd

Core Domains, Subcompetencies, and Description	Key Representative Concepts
Clinical data, clinical decision support, and informatics Searches, appraises, and applies information from literature and data sources to improve individual and population care; facilitates research to improve quality	Physician – patient level data; clinical- and system-level data Clinical data: research and quality improvement data Role of EHR data in exploring clinical and QI-based questions Artificial intelligence and machine learning Role of workflow analysis in optimizing use of clinical information systems Collaboration with data science team
Domain 6: Value-Based Care	**Concepts related to the performance of a health system as it relates to quality of care delivery, cost; from quality perspective, issues related to patient safety, effectiveness, patient-centeredness, timeliness, effectiveness, and equitability; from cost perspective, issues related to the cost of health care, waste components, and service requirements; also includes seeing and classifying gaps in care and care delivery**
High-value care, cost, and waste Provides patient-centered, high-value, cost-conscious care to individuals and populations of patients, specifically by integrating factors of high-value care into clinical practice	IOM dimensions of quality care (safe, timely, effective, efficient, equitable, patient-centered) Costs of health care delivery (inclusive of services required to perform health care delivery functions) Overuse, underuse (and misuse) Physician's responsibility for addressing value and costs (e.g., financial toxicity) Selecting tests and developing treatment plans that incorporate biomedical evidence, costs, risks, patient references Value-based payment Environmentally sustainable practices
Quality and patient safety Contributes to a safe culture focused on improving the quality of care and addressing systems vulnerabilities and failures as well as quality gaps	IOM dimensions of quality care (safe, timely, effective, efficient, equitable, patient-centered) Patient safety event reporting (including timely and effective communication regarding event) Epidemiology of medical error; error categorization or definition: active vs latent errors Types of medical errors (e.g., errors, near misses, lapses, mistakes, preventable); disclosure of errors Daily safety habits (e.g., universal precautions, handwashing) and personal responsibilities to contribute to safety culture Association between complexity in health care delivery processes and medical errors
Evaluation and metrics Uses data sources and recognizes limitations of data in health to assess for and provide value-based care Uses datasets and dashboards to seek informed practice-based feedback to improve patient and populations high-value care	Applying cost-effectiveness data to high-value care work Development and application of system and individual quality measures Core measures; PQRS

Continued

TABLE 2.4   Health Systems Science Competencies, Subcompetencies, and Key Concepts[a]—cont'd

Core Domains, Subcompetencies, and Description	Key Representative Concepts
Domain 7: Health System Improvement	**Concepts related to processes of identifying, analyzing, or implementing changes in policy, health care delivery, or any other function of the health care system to improve the performance of any component of the health care system. Issues herein include quantifying and closing gaps (action), variation and measurement (specifically related to quantifying and closing gaps, not to health care measures in general), analysis of data, and interventions**
Health care improvement Identifies and contributes to addressing systems issues to improve patient and population care	Variation and standardization: variation in process, practice; checklists, guidelines, and clinical pathways Operational excellence and high-reliability principles; Lean and Six Sigma principles Change management and improvement science; conceptual models of improvement Quality improvement tools (e.g., plan-do-study-act, Ishikawa diagrams, process maps, SIPOC graphs) Quality measures, including structure, process, outcome, and balancing measures; tools: run and control charts Human factors engineering – situational awareness Error analysis tools—error/near miss analysis; failure modes and effect analysis; morbidity and mortality review; root cause analysis Safety behavior and culture at the individual level: hierarchy of health care, flattening hierarchy, speak up to power; afraid to report, fear; psychological safety; closed-loop communication
Data and evaluation Uses data sources and recognizes limitations of data in health systems improvement	Using data to evaluate patient safety work or initiatives Quality measures Applying an equity lens to improvement processes via inclusive datasets and analysis

[a]Note competencies and concepts will evolve over time as new needs emerge.
EHR, Electronic health record; *EMTALA,* Emergency Medical Treatment and Labor Act; *IOM,* Institute of Medicine; *IPCC,* interprofessional collaborative care; *PQRS,* physician quality report system; *QI,* quality improvement; *SIPOC,* suppliers, inputs, process, outputs, customers.

ACKNOWLEDGEMENTS

Health Systems Science Competency Workgroup
The competencies were developed by the following group:

Jed Gonzalo, MSc, MD (Leader)	Penn State College of Medicine
Jeffrey Borkan, MD, PhD	The Warren Alpert Medical School of Brown University
Michael Dekhtyar, MEd	American Medical Association
Maya Hammoud, MD, MBA	American Medical Association and University of Michigan
William Hersh, MD	Oregon Health & Science University
Cindy Lai, MD	University of California, San Francisco
Luan Elizabeth Lawson, MD, MAEd	Eastern Carolina University
Joy Lewis, DO, PhD	A.T. Still University School of Osteopathic Medicine in Arizona
Kimberly D. Lomis, MD	American Medical Association
Pat O'Sullivan, EdD	University of California, San Francisco

Sally A. Santen, MD, PhD   Virginia Commonwealth University School of Medicine, University of Cincinnati College of Medicine, and the American Medical Association

Mamta Singh, MD, MS   Case Western Reserve University School of Medicine
Catherine Skae, MD   Montefiore Medical Center
W. Anderson Spickard, III, MD, MS   Vanderbilt University School of Medicine
Stephanie Starr, MD   Mayo Clinic Alix School of Medicine
Paul Weber   Rutgers Robert Wood Johnson Medical School

TAKE-HOME POINTS

1. HSS core competencies and associated key concepts can be used as a foundation for curriculum design and implementation for undergraduate medical education, graduate medical education, and interprofessional collaboration.
2. Core HSS competencies are expected to endure, but nuances of training and performance, particularly at the proficient and expert levels, must change to correspond with changes in the health system and the evolving needs of patients and communities.
3. Educational designers must implement purposeful assessment tools to ascertain competency development aligned with programmatic goals.

QUESTIONS FOR FURTHER THOUGHT

1. How do you integrate the HSS competencies into your curriculum?
2. How do you create assessments to demonstrate the achievement of these competencies?
3. Who would you engage from your institution's leadership as a collaborator to aid in implementing and assessing HSS competencies across the continuum?

Vignette

A newly appointed health systems science (HSS) director at a medical school is planning to develop and implement an HSS thread from the beginning of medical school until graduation. They plan to design the first 2 weeks of medical school as a boot camp for HSS to launch students into entering the profession. The medical school leadership fully supports this new initiative. Needs assessment demonstrates that students need to be competent in systems thinking to effectively implement HSS. The HSS director reviews the HSS competency table (Table 2.4) to determine what competencies are most important at this phase of training. In the process, they also decide to crosswalk the existing curriculum with the HSS domains and competency table.

Thought Questions

1. What process does the director utilize to determine the gaps in the curriculum, and what content is not covered?
2. How does the director determine how to sequence the content developmentally so that students are building skills?
3. What team-based activity or exercise can the director develop for the students to understand systems thinking and apply systems thinking tools?

ANNOTATED BIBLIOGRAPHY

Bodenheimer T, Sinsky C. From triple to quadruple aim: care of the patient requires care of the provider. *Ann Fam Med.* 2014;12(6):573-576.
This article recommends that the Triple Aim be expanded to a Quadruple Aim, adding the goal of improving the work life of health care providers, including clinicians and staff.
Borkan JM, Hammoud MM, Nelson E, et al. Health systems science education: the new post-Flexner professionalism for the 21st century. *Med Teach.* 2021;43(suppl 2):S25-S31.
This article proposes a framework for the 21st century physician that includes an expectation of new competency in health systems science, creating "systems citizens" who are effective stewards of the health care system.
Gonzalo JD, Haidet P, Papp KK, et al. Educating for the 21st-century health care system: an interdependent framework of basic, clinical, and systems sciences. *Acad Med.* 2017;92:35-39.
This perspective proposes an educational shift from a two-pillar framework to a three-pillar framework in which basic, clinical, and systems sciences are interdependent. The authors describe

the Systems Navigation Curriculum, currently implemented for all students at the Penn State College of Medicine, as an example of this three-pillar educational model.

Lucey CR. Medical education: part of the problem and part of the solution. *JAMA Intern Med.* 2013;173(17):1639-1643.

This special communication explains that educational redesign must begin with the understanding that the professional identities of physicians who were successful in the acute disease era of the 20th century will not be effective in the complex chronic disease era of the 21st century. It also advocates that medical schools and residency programs restructure their views of basic and clinical science and workplace learning to give equal emphasis to the science and skills needed to practice in and lead in complex systems.

Ridinger HA, Bonnet K, Schlundt DG, Tekian A, Riddle J, Lomis KD. Defining successful practice within health systems science among entering residents: a single-institution qualitative study of graduate medical education faculty observations. *Acad Med.* 2021;96(suppl 11):S126-S135.

In this article, the authors explore graduate medical education faculty observations of residents exemplifying successful practice across health systems science domains to inform targets for undergraduate medical education training and assessment.

REFERENCES

1. Lucey CR. Medical education: part of the problem and part of the solution. *JAMA Intern Med.* 2013;173(17):1639-1643.
2. Gonzalo JD, Haidet P, Papp KK, et al. Educating for the 21st-century health care system: an interdependent framework of basic, clinical, and systems sciences. *Acad Med.* 2017;92:35-39.
3. Combes JR, Arespacochaga E. *Lifelong Learning—Physician Competency Development.* Chicago, IL: American Hospital Association's Physician Leadership Forum; June 2012.
4. Gonzalo JD, Dekhtyar M, Starr SR, et al. Health systems science curricula in undergraduate medical education: identifying and defining a potential curricular framework. *Acad Med.* 2017; 92(1):123-131.
5. McGaghie WC. *Competency-Based Curriculum Development in Medical Education: An Introduction.* Geneva: World Health Organization; 1978.
6. Bodenheimer T, Sinsky C. From triple to quadruple aim: care of the patient requires care of the provider. *Ann Fam Med.* 2014;12(6):573-576.
7. Association of American Medical Colleges. *Core Entrustable Professional Activities for Entering Residency: Curriculum Developers' Guide.* Washington, DC: Association of American Medical Colleges; 2014.
8. Englander R, Cameron T, Ballard AJ, Dodge J, Bull J, Aschenbrener CA. Toward a common taxonomy of competency domains for the health professions and competencies for physicians. *Acad Med.* 2013;88:1088-1094.
9. Interprofessional Education Collaborative. *Core Competencies for Interprofessional Collaborative Practice.* <https://hsc.unm.edu/ipe/resources/ipec-2016-corecompetencies.pdf>; 2016 Accessed 19.02.20.
10. Institute for Healthcare Improvement. *Knowledge Domains for Health Professional Students Seeking Competency in The Continual Improvement and Innovation of Health Care.* <http://www.ihi.org/education/ihiopenschool/resources/Assets/Publications%20-%20EightKnowledgeDomainsforHealthProfessionalStudents_5216cd8e-1867-4c77-90b6-955641ecab78/KnowledgeDomains.pdf>; Accessed 19.02.20.
11. Association of American Medical Colleges. *Quality Improvement and Patient Safety Competencies.* <https://www.aamc.org/whatwe-do/mission-areas/medical-education/cbme/qips>; Accessed 19.02.20.
12. Liaison Committee on Medical Education. *Standards, Publications, & Notification Forms.* <http://lcme.org/publications>; Accessed 19.02.20.
13. United States Medical Licensing Examination. *USMLE Physician Tasks/Competencies.* <https://www.usmle.org/pdfs/ tcom.pdf>; 2019 Accessed 19.02.20.
14. United States Medical Licensing Examination. *Step 1: Content Outline and Specifications.* <https://www.usmle.org/step-1>; 11.03.20
15. Accreditation Council for Graduate Medical Education. *Outcomes Project.* <http://www.acgme.org/outcome/comp/compFull.asp>; 30.03.13. IPEC Core Competencies. Interprofessional Education Collaborative. https://www.ipecollaborative.org/ipec-core-competencies. Accessed July 8, 2022.
16. Guralnick S, Ludwig S, Englander R. Domain of competence: systems-based practice. *Acad Pediatr.* 2014;14(suppl 2): S70-S79.
17. Edgar L, Roberts S, Holmboe E. Milestones 2.0: a step forward. *J Grad Med Educ.* 2018;10:367-369.
18. Accreditation Council for Graduate Medical Education. *Common Program Requirements.* <https://www.acgme.org/WhatWe-Do/Accreditation/Common-ProgramRequirements>; 19.02.20.
19. Weiss KB, Bagian JP, Wagner R. CLER pathways to excellence: expectations for an optimal clinical learning environment (executive summary). *J Grad Med Educ.* 2014;6:610-611.
20. Institute for Healthcare Improvement. *IHI Open School Online Courses.* <http://app.ihi.org/lmsspa/#/6cb1c614-884b-43ef-9abdd90849f183d4>; Accessed 19.02.20.
21. American College of Physicians. *Newly Revised: Curriculum for Educators and Residents* (Version 4.0). <https://www.acponline.org/clinical-information/high-value-care/medical-educators-resources/newly-revised-curriculum-for-educators-and-residents-version-40. Accessed July 8, 2022.
22. Myers JS, Tess A, Glasheen JJ, et al. The quality and safety educators academy: fulfilling an unmet need for faculty development. *Am J Med Qual.* 2014;29:5-12.
23. Kasper J, Greene JA, Farmer PE, Jones DS. All health is global health, all medicine is social medicine: integrating the social sciences into the preclinical curriculum. *Acad Med.* 2016;91: 628-632.
24. Walsh DS, Lazorick S, Lawson L, et al. The Teachers of Quality Academy: evaluation of the effectiveness and impact of a health systems science training program. *Am J Med Qual.* 2019;34:36-44.
25. Starr SR, Reed DA, Essary A, et al. Science of health care delivery as a first step to advance undergraduate medical

education: a multiinstitutional collaboration. *Healthc (Amst).* 2017;5:98-104.

26. Starr SR, Agrwal N, Bryan MJ, et al. Science of health care delivery: an innovation in undergraduate medical education to meet society's needs. *Mayo Clin Proc Innov Qual Outcomes.* 2017;1:117-129.

27. Havyer RD, Norby SM, Leep Hunderfund AN, et al. Science of health care delivery milestones for undergraduate medical education. *BMC Med Educ.* 2017;17:145.

28. Patel MS, Davis MM, Lypson ML. Advancing medical education by teaching health policy. *N Engl J Med.* 2011;364: 695-697.

29. Patel MS, Lypson ML, Miller DD, Davis MM. A framework for evaluating student perceptions of health policy training in medical school. *Acad Med.* 2014;89:1375-1379.

30. Maeshiro R, Evans CH, Stanley JM, et al. Using the clinical prevention and population health curriculum framework to encourage curricular change. *Am J Prev Med.* 2011;40:232-244.

31. Harris D, Puskarz K, Golab C. Population health: curriculum framework for an emerging discipline. *Popul Health Manag.* 2016;19:39-45.

32. Veloski JJ, Barzansky B. Evaluation of the UME-21 initiative at 18 medical schools between 1999 and 2001. *Fam Med.* 2004;36:S138-S145.

33. Nash DB, Fabius RJ, Skoufalos A, Clarke J, Horowitz MR. *Population Health: Creating A Culture of Wellness.* 2nd ed. Burlington, MA: Jones & Bartlett Learning; 2016.

34. Wachter RM, Gupta K. *Understanding Patient Safety.* 3rd ed. New York: McGraw-Hill Education; 2018.

35. Moriates C, Arora V, Shah N. *Understanding Value-Based Healthcare.* New York: McGraw-Hill Education; 2015.

36. Skochelak SE, Hawkins RE, Lawson LE, Starr SR, Borkan J, Gonzalo JD. *Health Systems Science.* 1st ed. Philadelphia: Elsevier; 2016.

37. Ehrenfeld JM, Gonzalo JD. *Health Systems Science Review.* Philadelphia: Elsevier; 2019.

38. Gonzalo J, Chang A, Dekhtyar M, Starr S, Holmboe E, Wolpaw D. Health systems science in medical education: unifying the components to catalyze transformation. *Acad Med.* 2020;95:1362-1372.

39. Gonzalo JD, Dekhtyar M, Starr SR, et al. Health systems science curricula in undergraduate medical education. *Acad Med.* 2017;92(1):123-131.

40. Headrick LA, Baron RB, Pingleton SK, et al. *Teaching for Quality: Integrating Quality Improvement and Patient Safety Across The Continuum of Medical Education.* 2013. Available at:https://www.aamc.org/system/files/c/2/494316-teachingfor qualityintegratingqualityimprovementandpatientsafety.pdf>; Accessed 25.04.22.

41. Interprofessional Education Collaborative. *Core competencies for Interprofessional Collaborative Practice.* 2016. <https://hsc. unm.edu/ipe/resources/ipec-2016-core-competencies. pdf>; 2016 Accessed 25.04.22.

42. Association of American Medical Colleges. *Behavioral and Social Science Foundations for Future Physicians: Report of the*

Behavioral and Social Science Expert Panel. <https://www.aamc. org/system/files/d/1/271020-behavioralandsocialscience foundationsforfuturephysicians.pdf>; 2011 Accessed 25.04.22.

43. Moriates C, Dohan D, Spetz J, Sawaya GF. Defining competencies for education in health care value: recommendations from the University of California, San Francisco Center for Healthcare Value Training Initiative. *Acad Med.* 2015;90: 421-424.

44. Accreditation Council for Graduate Medical Education Annual Report. https://www.acgme.org/Portals/0/PDFs/an_ 1999AnnRep.pdf. Accessed July 8, 2022.

45. Gonzalo JD, Wolpaw DR, Cooney R, Mazotti L, Reilly JB, Wolpaw T. Evolving the systems-based practice competency in graduate medical education to meet patient needs in the 21st-century health care system. *Acad Med.* 2022;97(5): 655-661.

46. Batalden P, Leach D, Swing S, Dreyfus H, Dreyfus S. General competencies and accreditation in graduate medical education. *Health Aff (Millwood).* 2002;21(5):103-111.

47. Edgar L, Roberts S, Holmboe E. Milestones 2.0: a step forward. *J Grad Med Educ.* 2018;10(3):367-369.

48. Albanese MA, Mejicano G, Mullan P, Kokotailo P, Gruppen L. Defining characteristics of educational competencies. *Med Educ.* 2008;42(3):248-255.

49. Thomas PA, Kern DE, Hughes MT, Chen BY et al. *Curriculum Development for Medical Education: A Six-Step Approach.* Baltimore: Johns Hopkins University Press; 2022.

50. Skochelak S, Hammoud M, Lomis K, et al. *Health Systems Science.* 2nd ed. Philadelphia: Elsevier; 2020.

51. Plack MM, Goldman EF, Scott AR, et al. Systems thinking and systems-based practice across the health professions: an inquiry into definitions, teaching practices, and assessment. *Teach Learn Med.* 2017;30:242-254.

52. Meadows DH, Wright D. *Thinking in Systems: A Primer.* London: Chelsea Green Publishing; 2008.

53. Borkan JM, Hammoud MM, Nelson E, et al. Health systems science education: the new post-Flexner professionalism for the 21st century. *Med Teach.* 2021;43(suppl 2):S25-S31.

54. Ridinger HA, Bonnet K, Schlundt DG, Tekian A, Riddle J, Lomis KD. Defining successful practice within health systems science among entering residents: a single-institution qualitative study of graduate medical education faculty observations. *Acad Med.* 2021;96(suppl 11):S126-S135.

55. Dreyfus SE. *Four Models vs Human Situational Understanding: Inherent Limitations on the Modelling of Business Expertise, ref F49620-79-C-0063.* USAF Office of Scientific Research; 1981. Wright-Patterson Air Force Base, Ohio

56. Dreyfus HL, Dreyfus SE. Putting computers in their proper place: analysis versus intuition in the classroom. In: Sloan D, ed. *The Computer in Education: A Critical Perspective.* Columbia, New York: Teachers' College Press; 1984.

57. Association of American Medical Colleges. *Competencies Across the Learning Continuum Series.* 2020. <https://www.aamc.org/ what-we-do/mission-areas/medical-education/cbme/compe-tency>; Accessed 25.04.22.

Health Systems Science Implementation in Pre-clerkship Curricula

Karen E. Segerson, Peter Weir, Earla J. White, and Jennifer Meka

LEARNING OBJECTIVES

1. Explore health systems science (HSS) curriculum implementation in the pre-clerkship realm.
2. Apply an improvement methodology to the implementation of novel HSS pre-clerkship curriculum within institutions.
3. Describe educational strategies designed to enhance master adaptive learning to achieve phased goals and objectives.

4. Propose strategies for curriculum implementation and integration into existing or novel pre-clerkship structures as well as interprofessional, experiential learning opportunities.
5. Illustrate measures for student assessment of learning, as well as student, faculty, and institutional evaluations of the pre-clerkship curriculum.

CHAPTER OUTLINE

Chapter Summary, 35
Introduction, 36
The Relevance of Health Systems Science for Master
   Adaptive Learners, 36
Approach to Pre-clerkship Curriculum, 36
Pre-clerkship Health Systems Science Curriculum
   Development, 36
The Tactics (Organizational and Educational
   Strategies), 41
   Self-directed Learning, 41

Active Learning, 42
Collaborative Learning, 42
Integration and Implementation, 43
Evaluation of the Pre-clerkship Curriculum, 44
Common Challenges, 46
Conclusion, 46
Take-Home Points, 47
Questions for Further Thought, 48

CHAPTER SUMMARY

This chapter provides an overview of strategies for pre-clerkship health systems science (HSS) curriculum development and implementation. Historically, medical schools have begun with 2 years of classroom "pre-clinical" learning followed by 2 years of clinical training, the two-pillar model. Numerous institutions are evolving to move away from the two-pillar model and to integrate early clinical experiences and HSS education into the pre-clerkship years. The approach to development of a pre-clerkship HSS curriculum that we describe in this chapter follows Kotter's change management process, described in Chapter 1, and the model for improvement's Plan-Do-Study Act (PDSA) cycle of continuous improvement for making changes to the existing implicit and explicit HSS curriculum within an institution.[1]

We begin by examining the current system and crafting a vision for curricular content. Our process proceeds in developing phased-goals and objectives for the pre-clerkship experience. Planning takes into consideration varied learner experiences and uses the strategies of master adaptive learning. We provide examples of educational strategies linked with assessments. We describe the utility of measuring curriculum implementation outcomes and processes, with examples of how feedback on implementation may drive continuous quality improvement. We suggest strategies for implementation that draw from approaches of systems thinking as we broadly consider stakeholder engagement and partnership.

INTRODUCTION

Health systems science learning in the **pre-clerkship** years lays the foundation for advancing professional identity development and **systems citizenship**, with preparedness for systems learning and successful functioning in the 21st century clinical environment. Stakeholder investment in HSS by medical schools and their affiliated health systems is a prerequisite for integration with basic and clinical sciences in the pre-clerkship curriculum.[2-4] Community partnerships with health and human service organizations are essential for enriched HSS experiential learning opportunities that align with endeavors to improve patient and community health.[5,6]

THE RELEVANCE OF HEALTH SYSTEMS SCIENCE FOR MASTER ADAPTIVE LEARNERS

Future physicians are faced with a rapidly changing landscape in their work environment and with constantly advancing and adjusting medical knowledge. To cope and thrive in their professions, they must become expert, lifelong, flexible learners. The first book in the American Medical Association's (AMA's) MedEd Innovation Series, *The Master Adaptive Learner*, demonstrates the AMA's commitment "to assist physicians in becoming **master adaptive learners**—expert, self-directed, self-regulated, and lifelong workplace learners."[5] It is nearly impossible to predict what the health system will look like in the future, much less the medical knowledge and skills necessary to thrive in this environment. The Master Adaptive Learner Framework for how to adapt to change and remain lifelong learners outlines the skills essential to flourish.[6]

As referenced later in this chapter, relevance is one of the most important factors for adult learners. For future physicians, there may be nothing more relevant than the need for health care system reform. The US health system consistently fails to compete well with any country in the world in terms of health outcomes for the amount of money spent. Many future physicians, when prompted, can easily list the shortcomings of their local health systems such as health care inequities, failure to measure and achieve favorable patient-centered outcomes, and gaps in transitions of care.[6] Because HSS focuses on how health care is delivered, there is no better body of knowledge or skills more relevant for addressing these core issues.[6]

APPROACH TO PRE-CLERKSHIP CURRICULUM

Following pre-implementation steps of the Kotter model as described in Chapter 1, we recommend a systematic educational approach for successful curricular development, implementation, and assessment of pre-clerkship curriculum.[4,7,8] The purposeful application of **systems thinking** and continuous quality improvement philosophies, mindsets, and tools have proven useful to guide development, transformation, and goal attainment in medical education.[4,7] Through the lens of systems thinking, the big picture as well as multiple interdependent components of curricular revision come into view, with an intensified focus on how to bring about desired curricular revision. *How* to bring about change is as important as *what* to change. We include **implementation science** methodology in practical frameworks[9] to incorporate HSS in the pre-clerkship curriculum.

Understanding an institution's current state of existing HSS pre-clerkship curriculum is an important initial step to curriculum development, as explained in Chapter 1. This step involves detailing existing student outcomes, content areas, teaching and learning methods, assessment,[8] and learning environments.[4] Curriculum development teams may benefit from the Association of American Medical Colleges and the American Association of Colleges of Osteopathic Medicine shared Curriculum Inventory Resources.[10]

Following an inventory of the institution's pre-clerkship existing conditions of the HSS curriculum (Fig. 3.1), the curriculum team should advance with a systematic educational improvement process. In *Curriculum Development for Medical Education: A Six-Step Approach, curriculum* is defined as "a planned educational experience."[8] As depicted in Chapter 1, Fig. 1.1, the Kotter change management model is synthesized with the Kern model, which is also known as the six-step approach to curriculum development. The six-step approach is a practical evidence-based process framework to develop, implement, evaluate, and continuously improve educational experiences.[8] An example of the application of this approach to the development of a curriculum for **professional identity formation** is provided in Box 3.1.

PRE-CLERKSHIP HEALTH SYSTEMS SCIENCE CURRICULUM DEVELOPMENT

The initial needs assessment begins with an institutional resource scan to identify the state of the existing HSS pre-clerkship curriculum, and a needs assessment further seeks to understand learner stages, knowledge gaps, and the diversity of experiences of learners. Assessing the needs of the learners may be achieved in multiple ways. Surveys,

Student and Program Outcomes	Content Areas	Teaching and Learning Methods	Assessments	Learning Environments
• Understand patient-centered care • Use population- and community-oriented approaches to care	• Professional identity formation • Social determinants of health	• Self-directed learning • Workshops	• Multiple-choice questions • Portfolio-based assessment	• Classroom • Health systems

Fig. 3.1 Example institution's pre-clerkship existing conditions of health systems science curriculum.

BOX 3.1 Example Six-Step Approach to Pre-clerkship Health Systems Science Innovative Educational Experiences—Designed, Implemented, and Facilitated—by the Undergraduate Medical Education Department at A.T. Still University School of Osteopathic Medicine in Arizona

Step 1—Problem Identification

A literature review reveals urgency to broaden the scope and advance professional identity formation among medical students in preparation for engagement in health systems science (HSS) domains within complex environments.

Current Approach: Learners enter medical school with a general awareness of professionalism but lack comprehensive knowledge of professional identity formation.

Ideal Approach: Learners demonstrate an understanding of, appreciation for, and self-progression in professional identity formation in preparation for engaging in HSS in pre-clerkship and clerkship environments.

Step 2—Needs Assessment

A guiding coalition determines what learners need to know at what stages in pre-clerkship training.

Year 1 Orientation: Learners need to demonstrate independent and team-oriented awareness of professional identity formation.

Pre-clerkship Year 1: Learners need to begin forming professional identities.

Pre-clerkship Year 2: Learners need to apply professional identity virtues and skills in case-based instruction and learning activities.

Step 3—Goals and Objectives

A shared vision sets aims for learning.

Year 1 Orientation: Learners will develop and communicate goals for professional identity formation as individuals, as teams, and as a medical school class.

Pre-clerkship Year 1: Learners will begin forming professional identities at the onset of the White Coat Ceremony and through a series of HSS workshops integrated into four 10-week courses.

Pre-clerkship Year 2: Learners will apply professional identity virtues and skills in case-based instruction and learning activities.

Step 4—Educational Strategies

Using the shared vision, strategies are developed to achieve goals.

New Student Orientation: Small-group discussion and team-building activities (virtual, campus classroom, or student-selected locations): Learners are placed into teams of 8 to 10 members. After a brief dean-led introduction to learning in medical school and professional identity formation, each team collaboratively creates one PowerPoint slide to demonstrate what professional identity formation means to them as individual learners and as a team. All team slides are collected and placed on one class poster, which is displayed in a prominent campus hallway throughout the year.

Each team collaborates to develop a 3- to 5-minute audiovisual recording. All team members contribute their voice to communicate goals and key points for professional identity formation in medical school. This project generates a great deal of enthusiasm and camaraderie as the voices of all 162 classmates are heard in the orientation team video presentations to the class, administration, faculty, and staff. Team videos are stored in a Microsoft Teams HSS channel for convenient access by all class members.

Pre-clerkship Year 1: Large-group discussion and team-based activities in 2-hour workshops via virtual Microsoft Teams: The learner's responsibility for a broadened scope of professional identity formation is sealed with the Osteopathic Pledge of Commitment at the White Coat Ceremony. The professional identity formation theme is carried

Continued

BOX 3.1   **Example Six-Step Approach to Pre-clerkship Health Systems Science Innovative Educational Experiences—Designed, Implemented, and Facilitated—by the Undergraduate Medical Education Department at A.T. Still University School of Osteopathic Medicine in Arizona—cont'd**

forward in a series of HSS workshops integrated into four 10-week courses. Learners continue with their orientation-established professional identity formation goals and advance to health systems science domains that align with the biomechanical and behavioral-psychosocial models of osteopathic medicine. Each workshop begins with a brief large-group discussion and progresses to team-based activities in Microsoft Teams channels.

Pre-clerkship Year 2: Second-year student cohorts at A.T. Still University School of Osteopathic Medicine in Arizona advance to clinical learning environments within 17 community health centers located in medically underserved areas across the nation. This innovative approach provides learners with early insights into service gaps and areas for improvement in health systems. Students demonstrate professional identity growth through the planning, development, and implementation of service-based innovations that address one or more HSS domains. All 17 cohorts are encouraged to submit their HSS initiative to the American Medical Association Accelerating Change in Medical Education Health Systems Science Student, Resident, and Fellow Impact Challenge.

Pre-clerkship Years 1 and 2: HSS team deliverables are stored in Microsoft Teams channels for immediate and

future electronic portfolio presentation, which learners may also access in clerkship and residency years.

Step 5—Implementation
The pre-clerkship HSS curriculum is aligned with national benchmarks, accreditation standards, and programmatic as well as health center objectives to create short-term process achievements.

Communication of the shared vision and early successes empowers ongoing broad-based action to overcome barriers. This ensures continued faculty collaboration in facilitating learning sessions.

Step 6—Evaluation and Feedback
Gains are consolidated, and new approaches reinforced.

Learner evaluation is accomplished through HSS project deliverables and multiple-choice questions integrated into course assessments. Learner feedback is invited through workshop and course surveys. Program evaluation is assessed through institutional surveys, curricular mapping, and gap analyses. The quality improvement cycle following the six-step approach is continuously repeated to prioritize areas for improvement while acknowledging curricular gaps.

historical testing performance (e.g., United States Medical Licensing Examination [USMLE]), clerkship faculty assessment of entering clerkship readiness, and in-class assessments of knowledge and attitudes can greatly shape objectives. Many educators spend the bulk of their preparation on content, yet equal emphasis should be placed on the needs assessment, learning objectives, and teaching methods.

After learner needs are assessed, educational pyramids, such as those in Fig. 3.2, may assist in curriculum development by conceptualizing methods to progress learning.[11] These frameworks help in decision-making to align goals and objectives of the curriculum with educational methods, modalities, and assessments. Planning related to assessments and overall evaluation should be included in the initial designing phases of a new curriculum. As institutions or individuals begin their curriculum objectives, methods, and assessment planning, these educational pyramids help organize learning progressions.

The commonly used educational pyramids summarized in Fig. 3.2 include **Bloom's Taxonomy** to target educational objectives and assess progression in cognitive

learning, **Miller's pyramid** to target behaviors and performance and assess progression in clinical skills, and **Kirkpatrick's training evaluation** to provide programmatic feedback and assess the impact of the program on students and the patients they serve.[11] Assessments are described in detail in Chapter 7. Applications of Bloom's Taxonomy and Miller's pyramid to the pre-clerkship curriculum are provided here. Application of Kirkpatrick's training evaluation to the pre-clerkship curriculum is detailed in the section on programmatic evaluation, later in this chapter.

Faculty should consider the following example of teaching pre-clerkship medical students about chronic kidney disease (CKD) while connecting needs, objectives, and teaching methods in Table 3.1. The curriculum may first focus on cognitive learning progression. A student would progress through a number of learning objectives at the base of Bloom's Taxonomy before approaching the highest level of thinking. For example, before a student could apply a risk stratification model to a patient population to determine who is at risk of progressing to renal failure, they would first need to understand the different stages of CKD, and what

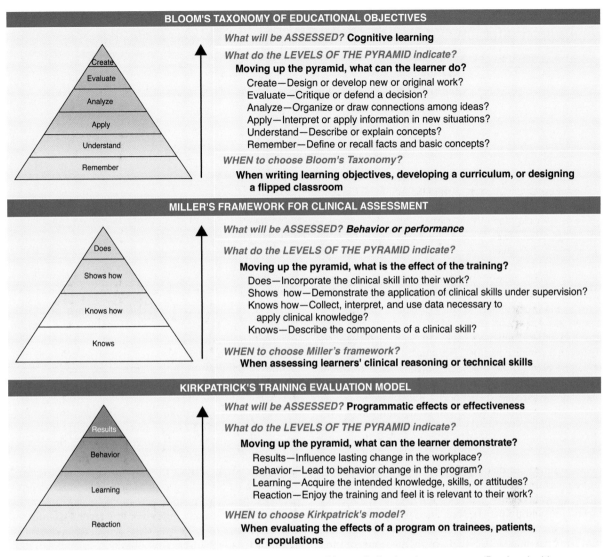

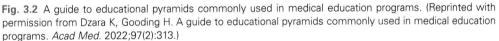

Fig. 3.2 A guide to educational pyramids commonly used in medical education programs. (Reprinted with permission from Dzara K, Gooding H. A guide to educational pyramids commonly used in medical education programs. *Acad Med.* 2022;97(2):313.)

clinical data points are used in that calculation. Likewise, a student would have to understand how risk stratification models are built (e.g., kidney function is estimated using the CKD-Epidemiology Collaboration [CKD-EPI] calculation) to explain how race and ethnicity bias in a health system can lead to disparate outcomes for Black patients with CKD. (The CKD-EPI calculation uses a correction for Black patients that may underestimate their degree of kidney function, leading to decreased access to services and ultimately poorer outcomes.)

After educational objectives have been created to progress cognitive learning, the pre-clerkship curriculum must also consider behaviors necessary to prepare the student for the clerkship curriculum. Curriculum developers may use Miller's pyramid as a framework for assessing clinical competence and to assist clinical educators in aligning their learning outcomes—or desired clinical competency—with expectations of what the learner should be able to do at any stage. Continuing with the CKD example, the student would

TABLE 3.1 Example Using Bloom's Taxonomy for the Teaching of Chronic Kidney Disease (CKD) Through Health Systems Science Lens

Bloom's Taxonomy	Examples for the Case of Chronic Kidney Disease
Remember	**Describe** the stages of CKD.
Understand	**Summarize** the risk factors associated with progression of CKD.
Apply	**Construct** a risk stratification model to determine which patients will have the highest risk of progressing to kidney failure.
Analyze	**Explain** how race and ethnicity bias and discrimination in a health system may lead to worse outcomes for Black patients with CKD.
Evaluate	**Rank** efficacy of established care models in achieving clinical outcomes for diverse populations of patients.
Create	**Compose** a novel CKD care model that provides effective care within a health system to achieve optimal patient-centered outcomes for a population that has historically had limited access to or been underserved by the health system.

begin in the "knows" base of the pyramid to identify risk factors and social and structural determinants that may impact health outcomes, and consider how she may solicit history in a sensitive manner. The student then progresses to "knows how" to use that knowledge in the acquisition, analysis, and interpretation of data, and in developing a care plan for the CKD patient. The student would "show how" by demonstrating the integration of knowledge and skills into successful clinical performance when interacting with the patient and demonstrating communication of a plan with the patient. The top of the pyramid, "does," focuses on methods that provide an assessment of routine clinical performance. The student may contribute to a CKD care model that addresses inequity and provides quality care within a patient population historically underserved by the health system. A summary of the application of Miller's pyramid to HSS pre-clerkship assessment modalities is provided in Table 3.2.

As shown in Table 3.2 and detailed in Chapter 7, common methods of assessment, such as multiple-choice questions, case discussions, simulation exercises or activities, and **objective structured clinical examinations (OSCEs)** target various levels of Miller's pyramid and provide sufficient feedback to learner and faculty to co-create a plan for continued learning and growth. Institutions may also want to consider using other assessments including **narrative assessments, collaborative examinations**, the AMA Health Systems Science Learning Series module quizzes, and assessments embedded within the Institute for Healthcare Improvement Open School courses and certificate program,[12] as well as summative assessments such as customized National

Board of Medical Examiner (NBME) exams or NBME subject exams for HSS. The MedBiquitous Curriculum Inventory Standardized Vocabulary Subcommittee[13] created a useful table resource listing assessment modalities and format options and defining them.

These formats may be adapted to serve HSS assessment needs. For example, the Geisel School of Medicine at Dartmouth adapted a portfolio-based assessment for use in a Health, Society, and Professional course. Students work in teams with a quality improvement coach and project partner to analyze a system and make recommendations for improvement. An artifact from this project (e.g., proposed recommendations) along with student reflections on project participation are included in a portfolio to demonstrate achievement of course objectives.[14] A second example is the adaptation of the oral case presentation from its traditional SOAP (subjective, objective, assessment, and plan) format to include assessment of quality (exemplified by the SOAP-Q framework used at the University of Washington) or value (exemplified by the SOAP-V framework used by Penn State College of Medicine, Harvard Medical School, and Case Western Reserve University School of Medicine.)[15]

Transformational learning occurs when pre-clerkship students synthesize quality and value-based practices as an integral component of care delivery from the beginning of medical education (e.g., while first learning the oral case presentation) rather than tacking on systems thinking in later clerkship phases. Assessments like the adapted oral case presentation may demonstrate the extent to which transformational pre-clerkship learning has occurred and indicate clerkship readiness.

TABLE 3.2 Application of Miller's Pyramid to Health Systems Science Assessment Modality or Formats

Miller's Level	Health Systems Science Curriculum Area Example: Social and Structural Determinants of Health	Assessment Modality or Format Options
Knows (fact gathering)	Identify key social and structural determinants, and their impact on health and well-being.	Multiple-choice questions; open-ended or constructed response questions; key features examination; extended matching questions
Knows how (interpretation/application)	Identify social and structural determinants that may affect patients as well as ways to ask patients in a sensitive way about social and structural determinants that may be impacting their health and well-being.	Case-based discussion; concept maps of patient cases or vignettes; open-ended or constructed response questions; extended matching questions
Shows (demonstration of learning)	Ask patients in a sensitive manner about social and structural determinants that may be impacting their health and well-being.	Simulated patient exercise or observed structured clinical exams; patient case presentations; evidence-based medicine cases; video vignettes; oral examinations; passport or checklists; chart audits with reflections, and so on
Does (performance integrated into practice)	Ask patients in a sensitive way about social and structural determinants that may impact their health and well-being, and develop an appropriate plan based on those factors.	Direct observation of clinical encounters; modified mini-clinical examination (Mini-CEX); passports or checklists or logbooks; 360-degree evaluations from multiple stakeholders; simulated chart reviews; global assessment forms; workplace-based assessments that may be tied to the core entrustable professional activities described by the Association of American Medical Colleges and incorporate a social and structural determinants of health emphasis; chart audits with reflections, and so on

THE TACTICS (ORGANIZATIONAL AND EDUCATIONAL STRATEGIES)

Pre-clerkship curriculum development should use educational strategies based in the study of the methods and practice of teaching adult learners (learner-centered as opposed to teacher-centered).[16,17] For example, adult learners prefer to engage in **active learning**. Adults prefer to discuss and process knowledge as opposed to listening to a lecture.[5,6] Adults have a diversity of experience, and allowing them to use this experience to contextualize their learning not only uses more advanced thinking but also produces memorable learning, although **passive learning** is not irrelevant. When passive learning is needed, content may be delivered **asynchronously** (e.g., recorded content that can be viewed at a convenient time). Allowing adults to be self-directed in their learning and extending them the flexibility to learn through different modalities are other principles of adult learning.[5,6]

Table 3.3 consists of a summary of concepts to optimize adult learning.[5,6]

A helpful framework for considering teaching methods best suited to adult learners and for achievement of learning objectives is to consider the following three categories of approaches to learning: self-directed, active, and collaborative.[18]

Self-Directed Learning

Adult education specialist Knowles described self-directed learning as a "process in which individuals take the initiative . . . in diagnosing their learning needs, formulating learning goals, identifying human and material resources for learning, choosing and implementing appropriate learning strategies, and evaluating learning outcomes."[18] Notice that the steps adults take to be self-directed learners mirrors the framework suggested for educators to create an educational plan (needs assessment, learning objectives, teaching methods, and evaluation).

TABLE 3.3 Concepts to Optimize Adult Learning	
Active Learning	**Examples Include Discussion and Activities**
Alignment	Content should match learning outcomes
Problem-centric	Use problem-based learning
Experiential	Link learning with previous experience
Safe, inclusive environment	Acknowledge learner's experience and knowledge
Self-directed	Learners want to explore areas of interest and relevance
Intrinsic motivation	Link learning to knowledge or skills that learners seek
Relevance	The learning has to be connected to what learners perceive is necessary

To promote self-directed learning, teachers need to take on the role of a facilitator who encourages the process of allowing learners to take charge of their own learning.[4] The following is an example of how to leverage this teaching method:

Using publicly available health data, students set out to analyze health disparities in the state of Utah. Students utilized a website, the Public Health Indicator-Based Information System, that contains health indicators that quantify disparities of care (https://ibis.health.utah.gov/ibisph-view/indicator/index/Alphabetical.html). The students explored the website's hundreds of health indicators to find one they found "disturbing or surprising." The students then presented their findings to their peers, and explained what they found and why they focused on it. Students considered what type of change interventions could be deployed to reduce the health care disparity.

Rather than delivering a lecture on **health care inequities**, this particular teaching method supports self-directed learning as students set learning goals, engage in the learning process, and reflect on their learning outcomes. The teacher's role is to facilitate the process and create the forum for the learners to reveal their own learning needs and present their learning outcomes.[16]

Active Learning

Allowing adult learners to apply their own knowledge and experience not only creates engagement but also affords the teacher a means to assess knowledge and attitude. Discussion and **problem-based learning**, for example, are two teaching methods in which learners engage with one another and express their opinions, often shaped by their own experiences.

Discussion: This is an example of an effective way to use active discussion as a teaching method to communicate the relevance of HSS:

The teacher asks students to reflect on whether they or their family members or friends experienced a gap in care in their local health system. Often this elicits a range of

interesting experiences such as a lack of access to mental health care. The teacher can facilitate a discussion using an HSS approach such as why mental health care access is poor in the United States, the health consequences of poor access, and interventions to improve access and outcomes. The discussion allows learners in a group to engage and to offer opinions from their own perspective that reflect their own experience and knowledge.

Problem-Based Learning: Students can be given problems to work on in-person or asynchronously outside of the classroom. This method is particularly effective if the teacher can simulate the kind of problem the students will be faced with in the students' future careers. For example, this is an example of a problem-based assignment:

Students choose from a list of population health management initiatives posted or propose their own topic. They explore the topic using literature reviews, white papers, trade news, key informant interviews, or any other means. They evaluate and take a position in favor of or against the initiative, drawing on the principles and frameworks presented in the course. They then prepare and submit a 10-minute PowerPoint presentation. A brief Q&A follows each presentation.

Examples of population health management topics include:

- Single-payer health care,
- Integrating oral health into primary care, and
- Executive order on price transparency in health care.

Collaborative Learning

Teaming is a foundational domain for HSS. Collaborative learning is an educational method that fosters teamwork among adult learners. Learning how to work effectively in teams teaches foundational skills for future physicians such as leadership and improved coordination and communication. An example of how to reinforce the principles of teaming in an educational setting is to assemble students in small teams (5–10 students per team), have them work on a problem, and then report to the larger class. Before the class, the instructor asks the students to take a brief individual preference survey for working on a team. The instructor requests that students try taking on a role they wouldn't normally assume. By mixing roles, students gain insight into the importance of different roles team members can play and how that contributes to an effective team.

INTEGRATION AND IMPLEMENTATION

After content and methods have been conceptualized, a systems-thinking mindset will aid successful curriculum implementation.[19] Implementation and integration processes begin with developing a coalition of invested stakeholders, developing an understanding of the big picture and shared strategies, and engaging in change management as described in Chapter 1. A systems thinker recognizes the changes required in curricular implementation across the continuum while considering the application of relevant learning theories and conceptual frameworks to intended student pathways.

The systems-thinking curricular lead identifies, obtains, and leverages available administrative support to promote curriculum changes. Early stakeholder input helps team members craft a shared vision, agree on rationale, communicate aims seamlessly, and distinguish roles for curricular implementation. By recognizing the limitations of mental models depicting the manner in which content has traditionally been taught, team members synthesize these models with current realities and pathways for advancement. Curricular pilot programs and feedback from curricular successes promote new perspectives and may influence acceptance of changes.

A systems-savvy leader identifies collaborations with interprofessional groups connecting siloed systems to capitalize on combining resources and shared goals.[19] An example of this is an interprofessional patient safety **simulation** in which a multidisciplinary team enters a room filled with potential hazards. As team members recognize unsafe practices such as the presence of a disconnected yet hanging intravenous fluid line or patient instructions provided only in English without interpretation services offered, the team discovers the diverse roles, experiences, and perspectives of each profession. A second example may include a multidisciplinary error analysis conference, when one facilitator analyzes errors across interprofessional services. In both examples, interprofessional groups not only share resources, but they also establish a culture where safety goals are mutually supported, and diverse perspectives enhance learning. Interprofessional education is detailed in Chapter 6.

Integration with content experts representing disciplines of ethics, social and structural determinants of health, and equity enhance understanding of the social constructs of the health system and the curriculum studying it. Relationships between systems structures and the knowledge, attitudes, and behaviors the system fosters are best identified using a multidisciplinary approach. As an example, a multidisciplinary session on psychological safety may expose concerns about system behaviors creating unsafe conditions for members of certain professional groups. Consider a system culture with a tradition of strong deference to hierarchy and the physician in a power role. The session on psychological safety with a diverse student group could effectively identify these power dynamics and discuss strategies to mitigate hierarchy. A discussion of health inequity between racial groups may identify differences in student understanding about social and structural determinants of health, and a skilled facilitator may be a valuable partner in navigating critical dialogue without fragility. Communication of ideals may expose quality chasms, sparking the need for responsive attention to student concerns.

Beyond the foundational knowledge addressed with receptive educational methods, HSS curriculum benefits from infused clinical activity occurring during pre-clerkship phases. Early opportunities for experiential learning and social construction of knowledge take place throughout the pre-clerkship curriculum. Health system leadership integrates authentic experiences within the system as learning opportunities. Whether engaging in service-based learning, analyzing clinic flow, mapping a visit, or interpreting population health metrics from a clinic dashboard, the HSS curriculum immerses the learner within the system in authentic and multidirectional ways. Students rapidly transition from a passive learning role to a value-added role of contributing as system navigators and engineers.

A diverse curriculum team with broad stakeholder representation is equipped to predict potential failures of curricular implementation and clinical integration, as well as failure causes and effects. Although curricular goals are necessarily time bound and curriculum implementation often does resemble its Latin word root *currere* (to run or race the course), diligent consideration of curricular changes should precede implementation thereby protecting vested stakeholder support. Change management tools, such as **driver diagrams, change concepts,** and **failure mode and effect analysis**, strengthen proposed curricular changes and identify potential weaknesses.

Although ideal for planning, systemic educational improvement processes are not without challenges such as limited resources, adding new content into heavy academic loads, and aligning HSS curriculum with real-life scenarios related to complex delivery systems. An array of opportunities

---

BOX 3.2   Example Introducing Health Systems Science Content With Gaming Science Innovations

Evidence has demonstrated that gaming science innovations are effective teaching and learning tools to promote student engagement, systems thinking, and the ability to strategize in complex scenarios. Gaming science innovations offer safe learning environments for master adaptive learning techniques in which students can plan, learn, practice, assess, and adjust new skills to gain proficiency. A simple Internet search using key terms such as "free games for medical school students" results in an array of useful websites with innovative options.

Gaming science resource examples that are freely available and easy to adapt for pre-clerkship learning of specific and overlapping health systems science domains include:

Health systems improvement: Institute for Healthcare Improvement Open School
- Emergency Department Flow
- Health Care Scattergories
- The Paper Airplane Factory

Population, public, and social determinants of health: Centers for Disease Control and Prevention Foundation
- Health and Well-Being for All

Value in health care: Clinical Odyssey
- Prognosis: Your Diagnosis
- Clinical Sense

(Data from White EJ, Lewis JH, McCoy L. Gaming science innovations to integrate health systems science into medical education and practice. *Adv Med Educ Pract.* 2018;31(9):407-414.)

---

to address challenges and introduce learners to HSS are possible during early planning and "in-between" phases based upon the curricular delivery structure of a medical school as discussed in Chapter 1. A few examples of such opportunities include the following:

- Emphasize content related to HSS domains in existing courses or competencies
- Add questions related to HSS domains in case-based curriculum
- Develop an HSS student club
- Introduce HSS content with gaming science innovations (Box 3.2)[20]

EVALUATION OF THE PRE-CLERKSHIP CURRICULUM

Measures are helpful in tracking changes in any HSS curricular situation to determine their impact. Measures provide feedback on whether the new curriculum improves on the status quo. Chapter 7 details how HSS leaders may apply Donabedian's framework for measuring the quality of health care to measuring the quality of education interventions.[21,22] This section focuses on the use of assessment to evaluate the curriculum and training programs in the pre-clerkship setting.

While planning the HSS curriculum, it is helpful to define the programmatic **outcome measures** one hopes to achieve to allow for better alignment among the inputs to achieve the desired effects of curricular implementation. As alluded to earlier in this chapter, the Kirkpatrick training evaluation model is a well-known educational pyramid useful for analyzing and evaluating the outcomes of training

and educational programs.[11,23] Kirkpatrick's model takes into account various styles of educational activities and programming based on four levels of criteria: reaction, learning, impact, and results.[23] An example of its application to the pre-clerkship curriculum is detailed in Table 3.4.

Process measures are helpful in providing feedback during curriculum integration to determine whether the system is functioning as planned when curricular changes are implemented. Content mapping occurs early in the curriculum developmental process, drawing from sources including national board examination content, institutional programmatic objectives, and online resources such as the AMA Health Systems Science Learning Series. In monitoring and reporting progress, it may be helpful to measure the percent of foundational content that has been mapped to goals and objectives throughout the pre-clerkship phase. Subsequent process measures include the percentage of phased goals and objectives that have been successfully implemented with a specific educational strategy. A checklist of educational strategies targeting master adaptive learners may aid in applying these strategies to phased goals and objectives. Periodically auditing newly created curricular content by tallying categories of educational approaches used provides feedback on whether the content creation is achieving the aim of targeting adult learners. Process measures may be aggregated into a progress report for stakeholders to leverage available administrative support, demonstrate early curricular successes, and promote curriculum changes.

A challenge inherent in adding curriculum content is expansion of the medical student experience and increased demand on overcommitted faculty, students, and

TABLE 3.4	**Kirkpatrick's Model**
Reaction	The reaction level seeks to determine if the educational activity was relevant, meaningful, useful, engaging, and so on and may be administered to various stakeholders to collect sufficient evidence. For example, students, faculty, health care teams, health system partners, or leadership may indicate their satisfaction with the curriculum by rating student clerkship readiness related to health systems science. This is often measured through end of course/program/activity surveys.
Learning	At this level, we examine whether students acquire the intended knowledge, skills, attitude, confidence, and commitment to the intended learning objectives of the educational activity. This can be evaluated through both formal and informal methods and through pre- and postassessments. For example, faculty might administer a pre- and postassessment related to systems-thinking skills or teamwork, or a pre- and postassessment to determine student knowledge of health care system processes or quality improvement.
Impact	This level measures whether students were impacted by the learning, and if they're successful in applying what they learned. Examples may include clerkship faculty assessment of readiness to participate in health care teams, student performance on observed structured clinical exams, or successful completion of a quality improvement project.
Results	This level is often the most difficult to directly measure but seeks to determine if participants were truly impacted by the learning, and if they're applying what they learn as evidenced by behavior changes in the clinical learning environment. Examples may include demonstrated progressions to the Association of American Medical Colleges Entrustable Professional Activities for entering residency, accreditation standards, program plans, or overall health care system quality improvement initiatives.

(Data from Ardent Learning. What is the Kirkpatrick Model? Learn the 4 Levels of Evaluation. <https://www.ardentlearning.com/blog/what-is-the-kirkpatrick-model>; 2020 Accessed 19.02.20.)

administration. **Balancing measures** of cost (funding) for curriculum renewal and implementation as well as opportunity cost (student and faculty time commitment) may be helpful in assessing the value of newly implemented curriculum and drawing comparisons of value with existing curricular components. Balancing measures may also help identify areas for gleaned curricular efficiency, such as cost-sharing programs across interprofessional health education systems, **value stream mapping** student experiences, and batching faculty commitment during less demanding periods in the academic calendar. Although these approaches may be intuitive, measurement enhances the ability of the curricular lead to report on successful implementation.

Structural measures also demonstrate efficiency of implementation approaches. Examples of structural measures in the implementation of the pre-clerkship HSS curriculum may include the number of new partnerships achieved with community organizations (e.g., partnerships with federally qualified community health centers) or the number of clinical affiliations achieved (e.g., affiliation with a private network of rural health clinics). If the institution aims to cost or resource share across health professional schools, structural measures such as the number of interprofessional sessions created or the number of interprofessional students instructed per faculty unit may convey these efficiencies. Each of the above partnerships may influence curricular outcomes, but interim measurement promotes new perspectives and mental modeling of a novel curriculum to foster support during early implementation. Measurement of novel **value-added educational roles** for medical students may aid recruitment of affiliates and advance the mental model role of student from receptive learner to active provider.

To systematically evaluate the effectiveness of curriculum, it is important to "start with the end in mind" and identify for each goal or objective, possible outcomes and outputs that can illustrate impact of the curriculum, including its effectiveness in meeting its intended goals while also potentially identifying other benefits and outcomes. A **logic model** is a visual or graphic depiction that presents the shared relationships among the resources, activities, outputs, outcomes, and impact for a curriculum or program. It depicts the relationship between the educational activities and their intended results or impact. Using a logic model for planning at the onset of curricular design and

TABLE 3.5	Example Logic Model for Health Systems Science Curriculum Component			
Inputs	Activities	Outputs (Short Term)	Outcomes (Midterm)	Long-Term Outcome or Goal
Funding Course and curriculum thread lead time Faculty and small group facilitator time	Conduct longitudinal workshops and case-based learning series for students on health systems science domain or topic. Students participate in local health system activities or experiential learning. Students participate in quality improvement team projects (with residents).	Delivered ##[a] workshop and case-based learning series in pre-clerkship phase of curriculum. Students participate in at least ##[a] hours of experiential learning activities in the local health system. ##[a] faculty involved in teaching or facilitating in curriculum. ##[a] quality improvement projects initiated. ##[a] quality improvement projects completed and presented.	Increased knowledge of health systems science content areas Increased skills in systems thinking, teamwork, and leadership as evidenced by self-assessment, narrative feedback, clinical evaluations, and so on	Graduate learners who are clinical problem solvers equipped to adapt to and manage change in evolving clinical environment; improve local health care systems by student involvement and partnerships

[a]Depending on the scope and scale of the program, numbers may vary.

using the logic model throughout the planning and initial implementation can help with ensuring that sufficient data is collected and opportunities for continuous quality improvement are embraced throughout. An example logic model for an HSS pre-clerkship curriculum component is outlined in Table 3.5, and logic models are described in detail in Chapter 7.

As demonstrated in the sample logic model, multiple data points are crucial for effective and holistic review of the curriculum, which may include course evaluations, faculty evaluations, peer observation, student performance on various assessment activities, and other sources of student feedback, such as just-in-time feedback sessions or informal surveys.

COMMON CHALLENGES

There are several challenges in implementing an HSS curriculum during the pre-clerkship years, including the following:
- The current curriculum is overcommitted, and there is reluctance to add new content.
- Students and faculty do not recognize how HSS is relevant to their careers.
- The faculty are frustrated with the burden of incorporating new content into their well-established curriculum.
- Students complain they lack the time to learn additional content beyond what they are currently being taught.

- There are not enough faculty with an understanding of HSS, and the knowledge deficit contributes to discomfort in accepting or teaching the content.

Many of these challenges have common themes that can be approached constructively. First, curriculum leads should obtain high-level stakeholder support before adding additional content to the dizzying breadth of medical education. Second, when introducing HSS as the "third pillar" of medical education, curriculum leads should recognize the cultural shift involved and the incremental nature of cultural changes. Third, leads should demonstrate to students and faculty how HSS is relevant today and for their future careers to garner support. Last, leads must foster the successes of the **early adopters**—the faculty and students integrating HSS—because they can serve as exemplary champions.

CONCLUSION

This chapter is designed to assist curriculum leads in the quest to foster enthusiasm to push past initial, inevitable resistance that accompanies the introduction of novel material by using improvement methodologies. We began with strategies for identifying areas for improvement within the existing curriculum, focusing on the pre-clerkship space. Using best practice examples, this chapter aids in crafting a vision for curricular content. The chapter offers guidance for development of phased goals and objectives, taking into consideration differentiated learner experiences and strategies for master adaptive learning. The chapter establishes measures to gauge improvement in curricular outcomes and processes. We provide examples of curricular interventions along with strategies for implementation rooted in systems thinking and principles of change management. Finally, we describe how stakeholder engagement is fostered by sharing early implementation successes to generate support for ongoing intervention, driving for continuous quality improvement. This strategy of tackling the broad HSS curriculum through cycles of incremental change is an effective method for transformation and improvement of medical education.

TAKE-HOME POINTS

1. A pre-clerkship curriculum should synthesize learner and institutional expectations, clearly define pre-clerkship competencies, and identify phased goals and objectives.
2. Curriculum leads should create and implement educational strategies and instructional methods targeted appropriately for the master adaptive learner.
3. A positive learning environment is fostered by a systems-thinking approach, early collaboration with stakeholders, effective communication during implementation, and transparent integration of feedback.
4. Change management strategies enhance sustainability. Incremental changes create buy-in and gather support for expansion in scope and scale.

QUESTIONS FOR FURTHER THOUGHT

1. What curricular aim does the institution hope to achieve with this pre-clerkship curriculum revision?
2. How will progress toward curricular objectives be assessed?
3. How will the curriculum match learner expectations, offer differentiation for varied learner experiences, and create opportunities for self-direction?
4. What strategies will aid in coordinating and integrating pre-clerkship HSS teaching with HSS clerkship teaching to produce a comprehensive integrated curriculum?

VIGNETTE 1

Dr. Silo is the health systems science lead in an institution with regional medical campuses across a wide sociodemographic distribution. She holds meetings with the site directors twice monthly, proposing goals and objectives and seeking feedback from local leaders and regional experts. Quarterly meetings include representation from the curriculum office, student block leaders, and specialized content experts. Dr. Silo learns that the case example from a health policy session proposed by the main institution intersects with a politically charged recent event in one of the regional communities. Local faculty express concern with the session. One faculty member provides the name of a professor in the economics department with expertise within this content area.

Thought Questions
1. How are systems thought processes helpful when implementing curriculum in an environment with diverse stakeholders who may not share the same vision or motives?
2. What approaches may be helpful when encountering resistance to curriculum change?

VIGNETTE 2

Dr. N.O. Vate is the health systems science lead for his medical school that historically has been slow to incorporate adult learning theory into its curriculum. Because health systems science is new for his medical school, he uses the opportunity to showcase how to bring the principles of adult learning to life. Before implementation, he presents the new material to the curriculum committee and emphasizes not only the new content but also highlights innovative teaching methods that he has read about in the literature to better engage the learners. He uses an evaluation format that targets the levels of Miller's pyramid to better pinpoint his new curriculum's strengths and weaknesses. The student reaction is immediate. The students note that there is a genuine attempt to acknowledge their knowledge and diversity of experience. The course evaluation demonstrates high student engagement and serves as evidence the students effectively demonstrate their learning through case-based discussion.

Thought Questions

1. What are common barriers faced by medical schools struggling to incorporate the principles of adult learning into curricula?
2. What strategies and tactics could be used to address these barriers?

ANNOTATED BIBLIOGRAPHY

Cutrer WB, Miller B, Pusic MV, et al. Fostering the development of master adaptive learners: a conceptual model to guide skill acquisition in medical education. *Acad Med.* 2017;92(1):70-75.
This article describes the importance of continuous adaptation in developing physicians to navigate cycles of change occurring in health care. It focuses on the need to develop both the ability to function efficiently in existing systems while also developing the skills necessary to modify practices for continuous improvement and to innovate to address existing challenges. It describes a conceptual model of learning involving phases of planning, learning, assessing, and adjusting.

Singh MK, Gullett HL, Thomas PA. Using Kern's 6-step approach to integrate health systems science curricula into medical education. *Acad Med.* 2021;96(9):1282-1290.
This article describes a curricular framework for competencies from health systems science using Kern's six-step approach to curriculum development. It describes implementation of a module on improving health care delivery and novel coursework focusing on population and community health with a focus on health equity. It serves as an example of curriculum development promoting competencies in health systems improvement and community advocacy for undergraduate medical education learners.

Wong BM, Headrick LA. Application of continuous quality improvement to medical education. *Med Educ.* 2020;55:72-81.
This article describes how the application of continuous quality improvement can help medical education achieve its goals. It is rooted in W. Edward Deming's system of profound knowledge and describes how each domain is applicable in medical education. It demonstrates how quality improvement methods help educators achieve the goals of improving health systems.

REFERENCES

1. Kotter JP. *Leading Change.* Boston: Harvard Business Review Press; 2012.
2. Borkan JM, Hammoud MM, Nelson E, et al. Health systems science education: the new post-Flexner professionalism for the 21st century. *Med Teach.* 2021;43(suppl 2):S25-S31.
3. Gonzalo J, Baxley E, Borkan J, et al. Priority areas and potential solutions for successful integration and sustainment of health systems science in undergraduate medical education. *Acad Med.* 2017;92(1):63-69.
4. Singh MK, Gullett HL, Thomas PA. Using Kern's 6-step approach to integrate health systems science curricula into medical education. *Acad Med.* 2021;96(9):1282-1290.
5. Cutrer W, Pusic M, Gruppen L, Hammoud M. Santen S. *The Master Adaptive Learner: From the AMA MedEd Innovation Series.* Philadelphia: Elsevier; 2020.
6. Cutrer WB, Miller B, Pusic MV, et al. Fostering the development of master adaptive learners: a conceptual model to guide skill acquisition in medical education. *Acad Med.* 2017;92(1):70-75.
7. Wong BM, Headrick LA. Application of continuous quality improvement to medical education. *Med Educ.* 2020;55:72-81.
8. Thomas PA, Thomas DE, Kern DE, Hughes MT, Chen BY, eds. *Curriculum Development for Medical Education: A Six-Step Approach.* 3rd ed. Baltimore: Johns Hopkins University Press; 2016.
9. Eccles MP, Mittman BS. Welcome to implementation science. *Implement Sci.* 2006;1(1):1-3.
10. AAMC. *Curriculum Inventory.* Available at: https://www.aamc.org/what-we-do/mission-areas/medical-education/curriculum-inventory. Accessed April 11, 2022.
11. Dzara K, Gooding H. A guide to educational pyramids commonly used in medical education programs. *Acad Med.* 2022;97(2):313.
12. Institute for Healthcare Improvement. *Open School Online Courses.* Available at: http://www.ihi.org/education/IHIOpenSchool/Courses/Pages/OpenSchoolCertificates.aspx. Accessed April 11, 2022.
13. MedBiquitous Curriculum Inventory Working Group Standardized Vocabulary Subcommittee. *Curriculum Inventory Standardized Instructional and Assessment Methods and Resource Types.* Washington, DC: Association of American Medical Colleges; 2016.
14. Gonzalo JD, Ogrinc G. Health systems science: the "broccoli" of undergraduate medical education. *Acad Med.* 2019:94(10):1425-1432.
15. Moser EM, Huang GC, Packer CD, et al. SOAP-V: introducing a method to empower medical students to be change agents in bending the cost curve. *J Hosp Med.* 2016;11(3):217-220.

16. McCall RC, Padron K, Andrews C. Evidence-based instructional strategies for adult learners: a review of the literature. *Codex.* 2018;4(4):29-47. Available at: https://academicworks. cuny.edu/cgi/viewcontent.cgi?article=1048&context=bx_ pubs. Accessed April 11, 2022.

17. Schwartz M. *Engaging Adult Learners—Ryerson University.* Available at: https://www.ryerson.ca/content/dam/learning-teaching/teaching-resources/teach-a-course/engaging-adult-learners.pdf. Accessed April 11, 2022.

18. Forehand M. Bloom's taxonomy. In: Lombardi P, ed. *Instructional Methods, Strategies and Technologies to Meet the Needs of All Learners.* Available at: https://granite.pressbooks.pub/ teachingdiverselearners/chapter/blooms-taxonomy-2/. Accessed April 11, 2022.

19. Stanford N. *Habits of a Systems Thinker.* Naomi Stanford Organization Design. 2019. Available at: https://naomistanford. com/2019/02/07/habits-of-a-systems-thinker/. Accessed April 11, 2022.

20. White EJ, Lewis JH, McCoy L. Gaming science innovations to integrate health systems science into medical education and practice. *Adv Med Educ Pract.* 2018;31(9):407-414.

21. Donabedian A. The quality of care: how can it be assessed? *JAMA.* 1998;260(12):1743-1748.

22. Botma Y, Labuschagne M. Application of the Donabedian quality assurance approach in developing educational programme. *Innov Educ Teach Int.* 2019;56(3):363-372.

23. Ardent Learning. *What is the Kirkpatrick Model? Learn the 4 Levels of Evaluation.* February 19, 2020. Available at: https:// www.ardentlearning.com/blog/what-is-the-kirkpatrick-model. Accessed November 29, 2021.

Health Systems Science Implementation in the Clinical Learning Environment: Undergraduate Medical Education

Dimitrios Papanagnou, Shirin Shafazand, Meredith Volle, and Rani Nandiwada

LEARNING OBJECTIVES

1. Review strategies for curriculum development that implement health systems science (HSS) in the clinical learning environment (CLE) for learners in undergraduate medical education (UME) programs.
2. Identify opportunities for HSS curricular evaluation and learner assessment in the CLE.
3. Discuss case studies that highlight tiered levels of HSS implementation in the CLE.
4. Identify tangible, existing clinical opportunities medical educators can leverage to integrate value-added HSS experiences in an UME curriculum.

CHAPTER OUTLINE

Chapter Summary, 51
Clinical Implementation of Health Systems Science in Undergraduate Medical Education, 52
Getting Started: Early Implementation of Health Systems Science in the Clinical Learning Environment, 52
   Who? Consideration of Learners, 53
   What? Consideration of Content, 53
   Where? Consideration of the Specific Clinical Learning Environment, 53
   When? Consideration of Time and the Sequence of Training, 53
   How? Consideration of the Educational Modality Being Considered, 54
Opportunities for Health Systems Science Implementation: Additional Considerations, 54

Practical Considerations for Health Systems Science Integration: Examples in Practice, 56
Transitions of Care Example 1: Hospital Discharge and Insurance Barriers, 57
Transitions of Care Example 2: Outpatient Appointments and Diabetes Disparities, 57
Transitions of Care Example 3: Emergency Department Care and Opioid Use Disorder, 58
Opportunities for Advanced Clinical Integration of Health Systems Science into the Clinical Learning Environment, 58
Additional Advanced Learning Opportunities, 61
Learner and Program Evaluation, 62
Potential Challenges Educators Need to Consider, 62
Take-Home Points, 63
Questions for Further Thought, 63

CHAPTER SUMMARY

In this chapter, we review specific strategies to implement health systems science (HSS) into medical student clinical experiences (CEs) and discuss different levels of integration and institutional readiness. We highlight existing opportunities for medical educators who are just beginning to integrate HSS in their clinical curricula, as well as strategies that can help educators amplify HSS longitudinally in curricula that are more advanced with regards to HSS implementation. Using a competency-based framework, we review the assessment of learners of

HSS knowledge in the clinical setting. We also offer examples educators can use to evaluate programs that aim to integrate HSS concepts in the **clinical learning environment** (CLE).

CLINICAL IMPLEMENTATION OF HEALTH SYSTEMS SCIENCE IN UNDERGRADUATE MEDICAL EDUCATION

Health systems science is relevant to all specialties, health care providers, and systems, and is naturally integrated into the daily practice of medicine. Consequently, it is important to frame HSS for medical students so that they can make direct connections between what they learn early in their preclinical training, and what they observe in clinical practice while working in the CLE. This is particularly important because the formal curriculum of medical school and the hidden curriculum of the workplace often contradict one another. Medical students may experience cognitive dissonance when they compare what they were explicitly taught in formal curriculum with what is implicitly taught through observation of behaviors and attitudes in the CLE.[1] This can present a unique challenge for many educators who primarily rely on a formal curriculum that is rooted in the basic and clinical sciences to scaffold learning in the CLE. With careful planning and partnerships, however, HSS can be successfully integrated into the foundational clinical training of undergraduate medical education (UME). Faculty should, therefore, be equipped with the knowledge and skills to leverage concepts in HSS to guide student learning in clinical contexts.

One of the critical first steps in integrating HSS into a clinically based educational program is to establish with which of the HSS domains each **clinical experience** (CE) will intersect. It is also essential that educators consider the strengths and potential weaknesses each clinical environment can offer before crystallizing plans for the educational experience. Each clinical environment, course, and clerkship has the unique ability to exemplify HSS concepts, and each merits careful consideration before implementation in a curriculum. The design of the educational experience should consider which option(s) will best meet the desired goal and objectives and which clinical setting will highlight specific domains of interest. Decisions made by the educator may be informed by the area of faculty or educator experience, the availability of CEs that highlight relevant HSS domains, and the interdisciplinary and interprofessional team members with whom students will have the chance to interact. Educators will find that the clinical environment is replete with opportunities for value-added work in which students can be immersed. Although HSS concepts are ubiquitous in clinical practice, it is essential that educators take a methodical approach to the clinical integration of HSS in a medical education program. Equally as important, educators need to secure support from key stakeholders including educational leadership, as discussed in Chapter 1, to plan for successful program design and development and to ensure a standardized approach to HSS integration.

GETTING STARTED: EARLY IMPLEMENTATION OF HEALTH SYSTEMS SCIENCE IN THE CLINICAL LEARNING ENVIRONMENT

The clinical working environment is a complex learning environment.[2,3] Unlike pre-clerkship experiences, which typically take place in the classroom or in venues where educators have control over the forces that inform teaching and learning, the clinical workplace is dynamic, unpredictable, and often influenced by the hidden curriculum. With rotating schedules, competing clinical priorities, and external drivers of health care, educators aiming to integrate HSS teaching and learning should be mindful of the forces that govern this unique learning environment. It is for this very reason, however, that the CLE is well suited for training in HSS.

Exposure to HSS concepts during the clerkship years allows students to apply content they learned in the classroom to real-life CEs. Leveraging the CLE allows students to witness the intersection of HSS domains in a variety of clinical areas. They also have the opportunity to retrieve foundational knowledge and examine how it plays a role in the larger system. For example, they may encounter a patient who is readmitted to the hospital but without the knowledge of physician and hospital reimbursement, quality metrics, interdisciplinary teamwork, care incentives, and insurance coverage plans, students may not grasp the systems-level issues that influence patient care and how they might impact outcomes. Regardless of the HSS domain(s) of interest, educators should carefully plan HSS educational experiences because students may not have the requisite CEs and foundational knowledge for them to "see" the connections within the system. Educators also have the opportunity to focus on content students covered during preclinical coursework and identify where in the curriculum the CLE can strengthen training in HSS.

Educators beginning to consider formally integrating HSS training into clinical educational experiences have an array of opportunities from which to choose. HSS training opportunities may focus on the interprofessional care team, the social and structural determinants of health that impact patient care, value-based care, health technology, the policies that govern care delivery, or the processes by which care is delivered in a specific clinical environment. Given that these are only a sampling of opportunities for educational design, implementation of HSS in the CLE can be daunting for educators in the early stages of implementation. For this reason, it is critical that educators take an intentional approach to HSS implementation that considers learners, the content being taught, and the context in which the educational experience takes place.

Who? Consideration of Learners

Implementing HSS into a CE requires that educators critically consider the background and training of the medical student. Although it may be easy to dichotomize medical students entering the CLE by their year in training, student CEs differ significantly. Students entering an HSS educational experience may also have varied degrees of comfort with regards to navigating the clinical environment; this comfort can significantly impact their engagement with the HSS educational experience.

Similarly, students require varied levels of supervision and guidance as they immerse in training that introduces them to HSS content. For example, when discussing high-value care in the emergency department (ED), it is essential that students have a prerequisite understanding of how care is delivered in the ED, as well as the barriers that may come into play when aiming to apply value-based care delivery principles. Support structures must be built into the CE to ensure that students who require additional supervision and instruction are identified and accounted for.

What? Consideration of Content

As discussed previously, educators designing HSS CEs may choose from several content domains, including core, functional, foundational, and linking HSS domains.[4] Domains of interest should not only align with the goals and objectives of the educational experience itself but should also map to at least one of the **medical education program objectives** (MEPOs) of the medical education curriculum. Additionally, they should consider the overarching goals of the course or clerkship in which they are housed. For example, if an educator interested in designing an educational experience that introduces third-year medical students on an internal medicine clerkship to the ways in which the **clinical decision support** (CDS) tool of the electronic health record (EHR) can be used to mitigate adverse patient events (i.e., clinical informatics core functional domain), the educator should align this educational experience with a patient safety-related clerkship objective, as well as an MEPO (e.g., analyzing practice using quality-improvement methods).

Where? Consideration of the Specific Clinical Learning Environment

From the operating room to the pediatric ambulatory care center, medical educators have a variety of clinical environments in which HSS educational experiences can be implemented. After deciding on the goals and objectives of the experience, careful attention should be directed to determine what type of CLE would best align with the intended learning outcomes. Furthermore, several characteristics are specific to each CLE being considered, which can easily impact the educational experience. Some of these include the following:

- The level of learner supervision, depending on the supervisor-to-learner ratio.
- The availability of interprofessional staff members, which can impact the likelihood learners will be able to directly interact with team members from other health professions.
- The ability to interface with the EHR, which may be contingent on parameters of the clinician workspace or computer availability.
- The level of patient volume and acuity may also impact learning outcomes because cognitive load can distract both educators and learners in the clinical environment. Additionally, time that can be allocated by available faculty member(s) for either supervision or teaching may be further strained.

As an example, an educator interested in implementing a training program that prompts third-year medical students to consider value-based care interventions through engagement with the hospital EHR will likely require close faculty supervision, time for discussion and feedback, and student access to the medical record itself. Such an intervention may be best suited to a small outpatient practice, in contrast to a busy ED.

When? Consideration of Time and the Sequence of Training

The educational value of clinical HSS experiences will be impacted by the temporal location in which they come up in a curriculum. Analogous to **Bloom's Taxonomy** of the cognitive domain, a widely recognized tool for instructional design,[5] HSS experiences that are implemented later in the academic year have the opportunity to appropriately challenge students and immerse them in higher-order (i.e., more complex and more specific) problem-solving processes. Third- and fourth-year medical students will have worked in several clinical environments by the end of their respective academic year; this affords educators opportunities to design experiences that challenge students to reflect on HSS content areas from a variety of clinical contexts and apply lessons learned to solve more complex problems. In this vein, experiences in the latter half of the academic year have the potential to promote deeper learning with regards to HSS.

In no way should this consideration deter educators from implementing HSS early in the year; rather, this should be a reminder that educators will need to create additional support and scaffolding to students to ensure their learning. For example, an educational session that encourages students to reflect on systems thinking in a busy inpatient hospitalist service is best scheduled toward the end of the academic year after students have had the chance to think critically about the core functional and foundational domains of HSS.

How? Consideration of the Educational Modality Being Considered

In addition to considering learner needs, HSS content to be taught, and the context in which the educational experience will take place, educators need to consider possible approaches to instructional design. Bloom's Taxonomy may be helpful in framing the graduated increase in complexity and mastery between HSS instruction at different levels over the course of medical school training.[5] Having an organized set of objectives for the HSS session to be implemented will not only help educators plan the session, but also help educators design HSS experiences with teaching strategies that are best aligned for both instructional delivery and assessment. The educational modality chosen for the HSS experience should be intentional and prompt students to engage in both lower and higher levels of learning whether it is a lecture on medical reimbursement, a team-based design sprint on health system improvement, a simulation session on effective teamwork and communication, or a virtual self-paced module on the structural and social determinants of health.

OPPORTUNITIES FOR HEALTH SYSTEMS SCIENCE IMPLEMENTATION: ADDITIONAL CONSIDERATIONS

Educators beginning to consider implementation of HSS educational experiences in a curriculum will likely consider clinical clerkships (or clinical rotations) as a first starting point. This is a reasonable strategy because it represents the transition from pure knowledge to clinical practice. In this regard, students will become active members of the interprofessional health care team and will be exposed to and immersed in the delivery of supervised clinical care, individually and as part of the team. Ideally, clerkships provide a safe space for students to interface with patients. Students will be expected to routinely engage in patient interviews and data collection about their histories, including asking about the structural and social

determinants of health; performing examinations; reviewing patient-related clinical data; working with the medical records and other forms of health technology (e.g., telehealth services); participating in team discussions about value-based treatment decisions; and, essentially, being fully immersed in the health care system.

Medical students commonly rotate through several disciplines over the course of their clinical clerkships. These include internal medicine, family medicine, surgery, psychiatry, obstetrics and gynecology, pediatrics, and emergency medicine. Although there may be other clerkship opportunities for HSS integration, the aforementioned disciplines are commonly offered to students in medical schools across the United States in the form of clerkships or clinical rotations. Given the unique CLEs associated with each of these clerkships, there are opportunities for educators to link HSS concepts and learning objectives with the unique CEs students will encounter. Table 4.1 highlights examples of these opportunities.

George Engel emphasized that patient illness could manifest at several levels of patient- and system-related factors in addition to disease pathophysiology. Although all clerkships have the potential to offer holistic approaches to patient care, depending on the institution or timing of the clerkship, specific clerkships may be best suited to integrate the interpersonal, familial, and societal aspects of patient care into student training. Educators are most successful with identifying opportunities for integration of HSS topics in these clerkships, particularly if they are in the nascent stages of HSS curricular implementation.

To assist with identifying which CLEs represent optimal starting points for the clinical implementation of HSS, educators should conduct a SWOT (strengths, weaknesses, opportunities, threats) analysis of each clinical environment under consideration. A **SWOT analysis** can serve as an educational strategic plan to guide critical decisions in the early stages of training.[6] After it is completed, a SWOT analysis can inform high-value areas for implementation or may even uncover strategies to better implement HSS in the right CLE. For example, a SWOT analysis of the emergency medicine clerkship may reveal the strength of the role that information technology (IT) plays in the acute care setting and provide the opportunity for student engagement with the EHR. In this example, however, the educator should balance the CLE advantages with ED staffing shortages (weakness) and the impact this will have on adequate student supervision (threat). Ideally, educators can focus on leveraging strengths, addressing critical weaknesses (when needed), taking advantage of opportunities that are in alignment with goals and objectives, and mitigating threats that can compromise learning outcomes in their students.

TABLE 4.1 Health Systems Science Educational Opportunities for Clinical Clerkships

Clinical Clerkship	Health Systems Science Concept	Educational Activity
Emergency medicine	Clinical informatics and health technology	Requiring students to actively monitor the patients waiting to be seen in the ED and pay close attention to ESI in the EHR. Students should examine patients' ESIs and alert the team when a patient presents with a score designation of ESI 2. Over the course of the shift, students can post comments in the ED patient tracking board, updating the team on patients' clinical courses. Aside from ESI, students can periodically update the tracking board with critical information for the team as patients are waiting to be seen (e.g., medication reconciliation, recent admissions).
Family medicine	Systems thinking	Assigning students to interview patients who may have repeatedly missed scheduled outpatient visits and recommended laboratory testing. For each patient, students can be prompted to identify the barriers that may have been at play and develop mental models for both the patient and the care team to arrive at a plan that better addresses each patient's needs.
Internal medicine	Value in health care	Requiring students to routinely review daily laboratory testing and imaging that is ordered on inpatients on rounds. For each patient's work-up plan, students should also report the relative benefit, harm, and cost of testing to the rest of the care team.
Obstetrics and gynecology	Quality improvement	At the end of the clerkship, students could be required to reexamine a patient whose care they were involved in and examine the case from the lens of quality. In this example, students could be asked to submit a brief summary of the quality of care delivered to an obstetrics patient by applying the Donabedian model. Students could report on various quality measures (e.g., structural, process, balancing) and the patient experience.
Pediatrics	Team science	Students can participate in in situ pediatric resuscitation simulations with the rest of the interprofessional care team. During debriefings, students could be asked to reflect on interprofessional collaborative practice during the simulation. TeamSTEPPS concepts could also be linked to events that took place in the simulation. Students could also be prompted to submit a reflective paper at the end of the pediatrics clerkship that shares their experiences in being part of an interprofessional team and the steps they are working on to be a more productive team member.
Psychiatry	Health care structures and processes	During the psychiatry clerkship, students could be assigned patients who they would longitudinally follow after discharge. This may take the form of attending patient visits with care coordinators and social workers. Through this activity, students can step into the role of patient navigator to be able to better understand the complexity and connectedness of the health care system.

Continued

Clinical Clerkship	Health Systems Science Concept	Educational Activity
TABLE 4.1	**Health Systems Science Educational Opportunities for Clinical Clerkships—cont'd**	
Surgery	Structural and social determinants of health	During the outpatient surgical rotation, students can be asked to independently screen patients for structural and social determinants of health. Students can be provided with a screening tool that they would complete for each patient. To this effect, students could identify patients who may benefit from resources in order to maintain post surgery follow-up visits and those who may be flagged for expedited consultation with a social worker.

ED, Emergency department; *EHR,* electronic health record; *ESI,* emergency severity indices; *TeamSTEPPS,* Team Strategies and Tools to Enhance Performance and Patient Safety.

Equally as important as identifying a CLE with significant strengths is identifying a CLE with concerning threats, because these environments should be approached with caution in the early stages of implementation when minimal learner or program data are available. For example, if a desired learning goal is to prepare students for helping patients navigate the structural and social determinants of health in a family medicine outpatient practice, students may need to work closely with their interprofessional colleagues such as social work and community health workers. A SWOT analysis that identifies a CLE with minimal opportunities for interprofessional collaboration would not be desirable for this specific HSS goal.

As an extension to the SWOT analysis, educators in the nascent stages of HSS clinical integration are advised to collect an inventory of opportunities that exist for various CLEs and clerkships. By locating and mapping existing opportunities, educators can link curricular goals with discrete CEs that would complement training in HSS. Such an examination of opportunities may highlight the internal medicine clerkship as an opportunity to focus on interprofessional teamwork and collaboration or target the ED as a CLE where students can easily engage with IT. Collecting this information may prove useful when developing a more longitudinal, vertically aligned strategic plan for HSS integration in the clinical years of training.

PRACTICAL CONSIDERATIONS FOR HEALTH SYSTEMS SCIENCE INTEGRATION: EXAMPLES IN PRACTICE

One possible option to integrate HSS into a clinical educational experience is for an educator to identify specific content domains to discuss during specific time frames. Given that students are going to be heavily involved in patient care in the CLE under direct supervision, faculty have the ability to choose patient experiences that will illustrate specific HSS domains. Approaching patient experiences with intention through the lens of HSS can scaffold the clinical encounter by linking the experience to appropriate educational content, tools, and reflection. Over the course of their training, students could then be asked to keep track of patient experiences that link to HSS and longitudinally curate an HSS passport where they could document their experiences under specific HSS domains.

Another option is to deliberately distribute HSS training across clerkships by identifying which clerkships best showcase specific HSS domains and building a curriculum that addresses that domain within the clerkship itself. For example, bundled payment systems and diagnosis-related groups can be easily integrated into the orthopedic surgical rotation, which will house didactic content and teaching experiences over the course of the clerkship. This approach naturally allows faculty who are more experienced in HSS to contextualize the domains in a more meaningful and authentic way, and in the process may serve to ensure some standardization of content and delivery.

Formally integrating HSS into clinical training has the potential to expose the hidden curriculum, which takes place when there is dissonance from the CE students are immersed in relative to the educational content that is taught to them. One example that highlights the hidden curriculum is a hospital's effort to promote a patient discharge before noon. When it comes to patient discharge processes, the health system itself is at play in many different levels to promote patient progression, improve patient experience, address bed management flow, and mitigate patient length of stay. The expectations for patient discharge before noon easily frustrates medical teams tasked with navigating the discharge process. Working under this constraint threatens many of the essential systems-thinking habits, such as understanding the big picture, changing perspectives to increase understanding, identifying complex circular relationships, and resisting urges to make quick conclusions.

To better illustrate how a single CE can intersect with multiple HSS content domains, we examine transitions of care from the lens of systems thinking. Although each of the following three examples focus on transitions of care, we examine multiple HSS domains, further leveraging student CEs as value-added work that can ultimately improve patient care.

TRANSITIONS OF CARE EXAMPLE 1: HOSPITAL DISCHARGE AND INSURANCE BARRIERS

A hospital discharge crosslinks with almost every HSS domain as it represents an incredibly complex systems-level process. A systems-thinking approach is necessary to successfully discharge a patient, and consequently, this process is a ripe opportunity for a novice learner to witness the interconnectedness of the health system. Practices rooted in systems thinking require that the practitioner notices subtle relationships between cause and effect, understands the "big picture," is able to change perspectives, and considers the short- and long-term unintended consequences. There is a clear intersection of leadership; interdisciplinary teamwork; patients, families, and communities; structural and social determinants of health; health care structure; clinical informatics; and value in health care.

Tailoring clinical didactic teaching of a hospital discharge allows students to recognize how all of these aforementioned factors come into play during patient care. Value-added work for students can entail having them interact with social workers and case managers from day one of admission. Full participation on daily interdisciplinary rounds allows students to present their patient and synthesize information that changes constantly over the course of admission. Students can engage with caregivers during discharge planning and provide counseling to ensure adherence to discharge plans in order to better understand home health needs, insurance and financial barriers to medications, and help at home. All of these intersect with the situational context of social risk factors, writing patient- and family-facing discharge plans, and regular participation in medication reconciliation. For uninsured patients, having students engage meaningfully with both

the social work team and the patient to navigate this process is a prime learning opportunity.

TRANSITIONS OF CARE EXAMPLE 2: OUTPATIENT APPOINTMENTS AND DIABETES DISPARITIES

Leaving an endocrinology clinic appointment in the outpatient setting to go home, although not clearly labeled as such, represents a significant care transition for a patient living with type 2 diabetes mellitus, and yet another significant opportunity for value-added HSS educational experiences. Systems-thinking habits[4] are also applicable to this setting, as well as close observations of how elements within the system can change and impact patient care over time. With regards to HSS domains in this context, there are innumerable links between population health, structural and social determinants of health, teaming, advocacy, and value in care.

For value-added work in this setting, students can participate in the care of patients living with diabetes between outpatient visits, when they are not physically in the clinical setting. Many components of HSS occur after the patient has left the clinical setting, with patients facing challenges with implementing the care plans identified with their care team. The time and space between clinical visits, when care is still occurring outside of the examination room, is referred to as intervisit care. Students can help patients navigate complex next steps that are delineated after an office visit because this is from where many gaps in patient care emanate. In the outpatient setting, students can assist patients with navigating social risk factors to ensure access to affordable glycemic agents and apply motivational interviewing techniques to support lifestyle modifications for tight glycemic control. They can assist with scheduling appointments and helping to explain the costs of additional testing and imaging. Students can advocate for their patients by amplifying their voices. Having students engage with patients in intervisit care can shed light on some of the challenges patients experience and provide students with the opportunity to meaningfully engage in troubleshooting the system in collaboration with the patient. Through these experiences, students can learn more about which HSS domains apply to their patients living with chronic diseases and which ones require further consideration. From a population health standpoint, the use of clinical informatics can also help prompt students to think about health inequities when tackling the structural and social determinants of health that impact how patients live and manage common comorbidities such as diabetes.

TRANSITIONS OF CARE EXAMPLE 3: EMERGENCY DEPARTMENT CARE AND OPIOID USE DISORDER

Discharge from the ED represents a third transition in care that may serve as an additional HSS training opportunity. Systems-thinking habits that can be highlighted in this context include mental models and reconsidering premature closure on conclusions when treating patients in the acute care setting. Additional HSS domains that easily resonate with this specific CLE include interprofessional teamwork and leadership. A student working in the ED can assist with grassroots changes, such as working as a patient advocate and using trauma-informed care principles when working with patients with opioid use disorder.

OPPORTUNITIES FOR ADVANCED CLINICAL INTEGRATION OF HEALTH SYSTEMS SCIENCE INTO THE CLINICAL LEARNING ENVIRONMENT

Depending on the circumstances, there may be opportunities for educators to integrate HSS training experiences into the CLE by building on existing HSS training in a medical education program. For programs that have deliberately integrated HSS into a preclinical curriculum, educators can reexamine established goals and objectives of HSS programming covered during the preclinical years (e.g., lectures, patient panels, modules, clinical cases) and revisit goals and objectives from the context of specific CLEs. For example, at Sidney Kimmel Medical College (SKMC) at Thomas Jefferson University (Jefferson),[7] transitions in care are introduced to students in year 1, specifically when discussing challenges in caring for patients with congestive heart failure (CHF) during the cardiology block. In year 3, during the emergency medicine clerkship, students are reintroduced to challenges of treating patients with CHF as they critically evaluate patients who require readmission for inpatient treatment. The latter example allows educators to integrate higher-order problem solving (i.e., higher-order learning on Bloom's Taxonomy) for the same HSS content, leveraging the context of the CLE. Although students are likely to haphazardly revisit preclinical HSS learning objectives in the CLE, educators should take a more intentional, deliberate approach to integrate HSS content vertically and longitudinally in a medical education curriculum. Not only does this approach allow for a more organized approach to curricular implementation, but it also assists educators in identifying appropriate opportunities for workplace-based student assessments of HSS knowledge and application.

Although clerkships remain the cornerstone for implementation of HSS in the CLE, there are opportunities to better prepare students for the transition into the clinical environment during preclinical training. At SKMC, the CE program represents the practical portion of its HSS curriculum.[7,8] It places pre-clerkship students in clinical environments where they screen patients for structural and social determinants of health. Students work with their peers in small groups to learn about the broader context of health, including interprofessional teamwork. As they work with patients, they have the opportunity to identify and critically appraise community-based resources. Clinical settings are deliberately selected to allow students to interface with patients and understand the array of underlying social and environmental factors that impact health outcomes. Under the program, small teams of students work with clinical health workers, under the supervision of a faculty member, to actively participate in care delivery and reflect on the systems in place that can either optimize or deter health. The CE program primes students for additional HSS training opportunities that lie ahead in clerkships. Educators and curriculum developers may choose to consider similar preclinical immersion in the CLE to maximize the educational value of HSS training experiences later in the curriculum.

Regardless of where in the curriculum advanced HSS training experiences are integrated, educators should periodically reevaluate initial SWOT analyses for the respective CLEs being considered. Clinical environments are complex, dynamic systems. A change to any part within the system (e.g., supervision, patient volume, clinicians involved, physical space, the EHR, teams, and personnel) can significantly impact student learning outcomes. Consequently, the opportunities and threats a specific clinical environment offers its learners are subject to change. Similarly, educators also need to critically consider HSS-specific resources and activities that have the potential to influence the curriculum as a whole. For more advanced clinical HSS training program development, educators may benefit from the application of a logic model to inform their planning (Fig. 4.1).

The **logic model**, introduced in Chapter 3, is a conceptual tool that can be used for program planning, implementation, and evaluation.[9,10] It considers resources, planned activities, goals, and objectives of a specific intervention and challenges the educator to consider the linkages between a program's resources, activities, outputs, outcomes, and impact. For more advanced HSS clinical educational experiences that build on content presented earlier in a curriculum, a logic model may help clarify how all the components function together. The model is represented by four sequential components: inputs, activities,

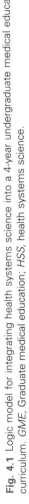

Inputs: what we invest

- Faculty with interest and/or experience in quality improvement, value-based care, evidence-based medicine, systems thinking, population health, public health, and leadership
- Mapping of existing opportunities within the health system where medical students can observe and practice important HSS domains (e.g. patient navigation, patient health education, improvement in process or outcome measures in various departments, health fairs, transitions of care, medico-legal partnerships, partnerships with existing nursing or social work programs, journal clubs, and wisely choosing campaigns)

Activities: what we do

- Develop and implement case-based learning that can be incorporated into identified experiential opportunities
- Develop and implement self-directed learning modules that introduce HSS domains

Identify introductory HSS concepts that can be included in pre-clerkship didactic sessions

Using curriculum map of existing opportunities, identify clinical learning experiences where one or more HSS domains can be practiced

Outputs: who we train

Undergraduate Medical Education (UME): Pre-clerkship, clerkship, and medical students in sub-internships

Opportunities to develop interdisciplinary sessions with medical students and other health fields (nursing, social work, public health, health administration/MBA students)

Opportunities to integrate certain experiences with graduate medical education (e.g. discuss value-based care and cost of services with residents and fourth year medical students in a general medicine rotation)

Outcomes

Short and long terms

- Robust foundational skills in HSS
- Student recognition of 21st century US health system challenges and their role in addressing these challenges

- Building team and system-level thinking skills through interdisciplinary opportunities

- Strengthened UME and GME connections using clinical experiences as opportunities to demonstrate and practice applied HSS domains

Measurements

- Student knowledge assessments
- Student satisfaction with didactic components of the program
- Evaluation of scholarly projects in mentored HSS domains (e.g. Quality improvement project)

- Observation of team interactions, and rating of team members
- Team project presentation

- Evaluation of student based on a prior defined goals (e.g. patient navigation: patient and student satisfaction with the navigation process will be evaluated, patient's appropriate use of health resources can be measured)

Impact

- Training physicians to address 21st century health challenges by practicing evidence-based, high-value caue; advocating effectively for patients, and communities; navigating health systems and organizational processes; shaping health policy, and leading change

Fig. 4.1 Logic model for integrating health systems science into a 4-year undergraduate medical education curriculum. *GME,* Graduate medical education; *HSS,* health systems science.

outputs, and outcomes. A fifth component—impact—has also been added to this model. Inputs and activities compose the planned work domain. Outputs and outcomes comprise the intended outcomes domain. By having a structural framework for designing clinical HSS experiences in mind, educators can better plan the intervention and better connect the experience with other related experiences within the curriculum. Furthermore, it may facilitate communication between all stakeholders involved in the educational program.

Case Study

In discussions with the clerkship directors of your medical school and encouraged by the dean who wants to transform medical education by supporting health systems science (HSS) content as an important third pillar of the undergraduate medical education curriculum, you recognize that many of your colleagues are teaching HSS topics throughout the curriculum, but their efforts are siloed and not well integrated across pre-clerkship and clerkship experiences. You decide to create a framework for an HSS program that spans all 4 years of medical school and builds on existing learning opportunities. You create a logic model (see Fig. 4.1) that summarizes program goals, assets, inputs, activities, outcomes, assessments, and overall impact. You present this logic model at the next joint pre-clerkship and clerkship directors meeting and ask your colleagues to help you map existing HSS learning opportunities throughout the curriculum. Armed with this curricular map and your knowledge of HSS core, linking, and cross-cutting domains, you recruit several interested faculty members to think through the other elements of the logic model and start creating a more integrated HSS curriculum in the clinical learning environment.

In addition to linking preclinical HSS content with educational experiences in the CLE, educators have the opportunity to design CEs that cross clerkships. Next we share examples from several medical schools that capture how HSS experiences can be designed to span one or more clinical clerkships.

The Perelman School of Medicine at the University of Pennsylvania has introduced an integrated approach to HSS training that begins with the Foundations of Health Systems Science Clinical Clerkship Correlation course. This course takes place immediately before students begin their clerkships and focuses on several clinical domains, including health inequities, innovations in health care, quality improvement and patient safety, telehealth, population health, high-value care, and insurance. In this course, students engage in thinking about systems problems through stakeholder interviews and tools, such as fishbone diagrams, 5 Whys diagrams, impact and feasibility mapping, and assumption maps to brainstorm interventions. At each session, students discuss how these skills could be applied to different clerkships. Students are then challenged to make commitments to action before beginning their clerkship for systems-based patient care.

The overarching goal is to create the lens for students to "see" HSS in action during their clerkships and to have a set of actionable items at the start of their clerkship experiences. These topics are then highlighted with HSS intersession days that are spread throughout the year, when the entire class convenes to take a closer examination into one of the topics they were introduced to in the Foundations course. For example, on the interdisciplinary team intersession, students interview multiple interdisciplinary team members in groups to establish best practices for working together. This is followed by group presentations to their peers about lessons learned and clinical pearls.

At the University of Miami, Miller School of Medicine (UMSOM), the NextGen curriculum incorporates teachings in HSS domains during small-group facilitated sessions.[11] Medicine as a Profession (MAP) is a longitudinal course that teaches students the essentials of medical practice and leadership skills throughout pre-clerkship and clerkship years.[12] Students work together in small groups, guided by a faculty member, to discuss cases that illustrate HSS topics such as professionalism, population health, wellness, ethics, and critical appraisal of the literature. Self-directed learning opportunities and multimedia-guided learning resources allow for a flipped-classroom approach where students come prepared to discuss cases and learn together as a team. In the pre-clerkship phase, students gain first-hand experience of the health system by serving as patient navigators, working at health fairs or federally qualified health centers to guide patients through the health system. Through this experience, students serve as active members of the care team. The MAP program continues in the CLE, in which clerkship students meet on a regular basis, regardless of which clerkship they are completing, to discuss their CEs and how they relate to HSS domains. Faculty facilitate these discussions and highlight themes that are common across all clerkships. Students are introduced to health care costs and quality concepts in the pre-clerkship phase and developmentally gain a better understanding of value-based care and quality improvement when it is reintroduced during clerkships. Facilitated case-based and small-group learning are also important elements of this curriculum.[12]

Southern Illinois University (SIU) School of Medicine offers an HSS curriculum that is facilitated by the

Department of Population Science and Policy.[13] After covering all core domains during the preclinical years, clerkship students are tasked with challenging the hidden curriculum to make connections between what they have learned in years 1 and 2 of training and the experiences they have had during their clinical clerkships. As an example, in the pediatrics clerkship, students receive a brief orientation that reviews population health and structural and social determinants of health and then explore how these considerations present in the CLE. Students are provided with population health examples appropriate for pediatrics including state, newborn metabolic and hearing screenings as well as critical congenital heart disease screening in the nursery; the Edinburgh Postpartum Depression Scale for sreenings in the outpatient clinic; Ages and Stages questionnaires; lead hemoglobin screenings for infants; and pediatric symptom checklists for young children and teenagers. HSS has a clear function in connecting preclinical knowledge with the clinical curriculum. HSS integration in the CLE can assist students with identifying and addressing issues that impact the health of the greater pediatric population. Although most students can define the structural and social determinants of health, this augmented clerkship experience provides higher-order learning and allows students to draw connections between infants' recurrent diaper dermatitis and families who must prioritize formula over the cost of disposable diapers. Although this example is specific to pediatrics, it can be extrapolated to any clerkship and helps students recognize similar HSS content across the clerkships.

ADDITIONAL ADVANCED LEARNING OPPORTUNITIES

Outside of pre-clerkship CEs and clerkship experiences, HSS can be integrated into advanced learning opportunities in the form of electives. Depending on the institution, there may be several policy, quality improvement, or patient safety senior electives that allow students to explore topics of their interests. One possible option is to simply rebrand existing electives from the lens of HSS so that students understand that they appropriately fit under this umbrella topic. Some programs have created HSS tracks or pathways in which students can create an experience of multiple electives and scholarly work that highlights a specific domain of their interest.

The Perelman School of Medicine at the University of Pennsylvania has developed a Frontiers in Primary Care and Health Systems Science elective.[14] In this elective, students gain exposure to advanced content on the health systems' innovation practices, quality improvement, and patient safety. For 2 weeks in the afternoons, they are immersed in a clinical site to engage in real-time observation, pilot testing, and interviewing through intensive contextual inquiry. This work has partnered with the Children's Hospital of Pennsylvania Possibility Project and the Penn Med Center for Health Care Innovation. These groups provide ongoing system-level projects that allow students to add value through these innovation sprints by being embedded in the clinical sites and continuing to work on their active projects

SIU School of Medicine also engages fourth-year students in electives that explore the intersections between HSS and medicine, an opportunity that allows students to consider how they will use their HSS knowledge as they prepare for residency. Electives, such as Population Health Leadership, Advancing Health Equity in Clinical Practice, and Cancer Health Disparities are available to all fourth-year students and offer a chance to tailor their experience to a specialty-specific area of interest.

Medical schools also have the opportunity to develop and curate longitudinal HSS specialty tracks over the course of medical school training. At the SKMC at Jefferson, for example, students have the opportunity to enroll in the Health Policy and Systems (HPS) track while being a matriculated medical student through the Scholarly Inquiry (SI) Program. SI is a required component of the curriculum and is intended to provide medical students with skills and experiences to become critical consumers and producers of medical knowledge. As part of an integrated curriculum, SI overlaps and complements training from a variety of curricular threads, including evidence-based medicine, HSS, professionalism and ethics, wellness, and the humanities threads. The HPS track was designed to advance students' ability to assess the effectiveness of current models of care, appreciate how health care is delivered, and understand the drivers that shape and guide public policy. This program, as well as similar longitudinal programs, fully immerses students in CEs that focus on skills development within leadership, patient safety, quality improvement, and IT.

Several medical schools have required students to complete a capstone, or scholarly project, before graduation. These projects are excellent opportunities for students to reflect on the applicability and relatedness of their scholarly work to HSS domains. This can be considered even in the context of a basic science project in which a foundational science finding will eventually have a human and population health application as well as economic implications. At UMSOM, students who do not participate in dual-degree programs choose from a variety of specialty pathway experiences (e.g., population health and policy, women's health, business of medicine, global surgery, clinical informatics).[11] A mentored scholarly project is an expected outcome from each of these pathways, culminating in a student day of oral and poster presentations. Students are required to consider and report how their project reflects an HSS theme or how it will impact the health system during these presentations. Similarly, at the SKMC at Jefferson, students are expected to complete a scholarly project for the SI program by the end of their second year, before beginning clinical clerkship. Students enrolled in the HPS track have an opportunity to focus their scholarly work on any of the HSS domains.

Finally, medical schools with access to schools of public or population health can facilitate educational pipelines to degree-granting programs whose coursework can complement HSS principles (e.g., master of public health [MPH]). At both the UMSOM and SKMC at Jefferson, students have the option of applying to a 4-year integrated dual-degree MD/MPH program.[8,11] After being accepted, students begin their MPH courses in their first year of medical school and continue with longitudinal courses that are incorporated into their medical training. MD/MPH students gain competency and experience in a variety of HSS domains including health policy, population health, evidence-based medicine, health economics, and health systems and processes.

LEARNER AND PROGRAM EVALUATION

The Association of American Medical College's 13 **core entrustable professional activities** (EPAs) for entering residency provide a framework for observing and assessing medical students' competencies as they progress through the UME curriculum.[15] Several of the EPAs discuss functions that reflect HSS core, linking, and cross-cutting domains (Fig. 1.2). For example, *EPA 3: Recommend and Interpret Common Screening and Diagnostic Tests,* discusses progression to observing entrustable behaviors across multiple clinical encounters where the medical student becomes competent at understanding the performance properties of screening and diagnostic tests (evidence-based medicine) and can order appropriate cost-effective tests (health care policy, economics, value-based care). *EPA 7: Form Clinical Questions and Retrieve Evidence to Advance Patient Care* highlights competencies in the application of evidence-based medicine principles. Knowledge checks on HSS topics, such as health system processes and critical appraisal of the literature, can be used to evaluate student mastery of facts during pre-clerkship didactic sessions. Throughout the CLE, there are many opportunities to observe student knowledge of and competency in performing various HSS-related domains. Educators should consider formative assessments that allow for opportunities to discuss HSS concepts and provide feedback on student application of these concepts (e.g., student approach to

choosing and communicating the most cost-effective treatment plan for a patient while considering patient wishes and best evidence).

It is important to consider and *incorporate* regular evaluations of HSS curricular content and incorporate learner and faculty feedback into program improvement.

POTENTIAL CHALLENGES EDUCATORS NEED TO CONSIDER

All changes to a curriculum come with unique challenges. Completing a SWOT analysis, described previously in this chapter, helps educators identify specific challenges to their program upfront and help them plan accordingly. One challenge educators need to address is how HSS topics should be integrated throughout the curriculum. Students are asked to become proficient in basic sciences in a short timeframe and then apply that knowledge to the CLE when they enter clerkships. Finding space in an existing curriculum that is traditionally heavy in basic sciences requires a carefully thought-out approach, but with strategic partnerships among the faculty and course directors it can be accomplished successfully.

In the pre-clinical years, one of the greatest perceived barriers is the availability of time in the curriculum. Just as professionalism, physical examination skills, and medical ethics are not confined to one body system, an HSS curriculum must occur concurrently throughout all preclinical and clinical years to provide training that is essential for future physicians. When HSS is presented as a thread, or streamer, along with other established content, it will negate the perception that it requires added time in the preclinical years and will also prepare students as they challenge the hidden curriculum once they enter the CLE. Making the connections early on between HSS and clinical practice can help students engage in clinical practice more effectively. In the same way that students learn how blood cell structure and altered genetic makeup can lead to sickle cell disease, for example, students can explore how systems barriers, structural and social determinants of health, and population health intersect with this blood disorder.

Another serious challenge to HSS implementation in the curriculum is faculty engagement in both the preclinical and clinical environments. Many basic science faculty members do not feel comfortable engaging in or teaching HSS material and may not have had explicit HSS training themselves. This should not be surprising. These faculty should be supported. With proper recognition and available support, this may be an opportunity to have students and faculty learn together simultaneously. SIU School of

Medicine's Department of Population Science and Policy addresses this in preclinical lectures, in which HSS topics are typically taught by a pair of faculty members, including one who is a subject expert and another who practices medicine clinically. This gives students the depth of content needed from faculty who are comfortable teaching the granular details and practitioners who provide a context for how to view HSS topics in the way students will interact with them in the future as physicians working in a complex health care system. At the SKMC at Jefferson, where case-based learning is used in the preclinical years, HSS cases are provided for faculty facilitators to prompt student dialogue for case-specific HSS discussions. Using patient panels to talk about their lived experience is another possible example of ways to address the hidden curriculum and help students engage with this content.

Buy-in from clinical faculty and residents is essential as well. Although students may formally receive HSS training in their preclinical years, if it is ignored when they enter clinical spaces, students may get the false impression that HSS is not prioritized or practiced by their physician colleagues. Therefore, it is necessary to help clinical preceptors recognize the many ways in which they already engage with HSS content in their practices. Peers in their specialties who can champion this work from within are an essential resource for HSS educators and curriculum designers. In fact, these individuals can also be consulted when building preclinical content and drawing connections to clinical practice.

After a plan for integrating HSS in the curriculum has been developed, it is important to include faculty development as part of the implementation process. Most faculty did not receive formal HSS training during medical school and therefore may have concerns about how to engage with

their students when discussing HSS topics, either in the preclinical setting or the CLE. Faculty development can help address these barriers and may potentially secure buy-in from faculty who will ultimately determine the success or failure of a program. This may require faculty training, protected time for training, time for teaching HSS, and practical examples in faculty guides that can be referred to when teaching in the CLE.

Learner assessment and providing formative feedback to students also play important roles during implementation of HSS training in the CLE. Faculty development should precede student assessment to address faculty comfort levels in both modeling and assessing HSS in the CLE. This highlights the importance of commitment and participation from stakeholders at the undergraduate and graduate medical education, as well as departmental levels. Other important stakeholders to consider at the institution are the dean, department chair, and clerkship directors. One may use **Liaison Committee on Medical Education** goals to demonstrate how an HSS curriculum is meeting individual departmental needs. Clerkship directors have ever-growing challenges and crafting specialty-specific connections to HSS may help them meet their own goals as well.

Educators have several strategies available to them to implement HSS into medical student CEs depending on the desired level of integration and institutional readiness. In this chapter, we have shared opportunities for medical educators to integrate HSS in their clinical educational programs. With intentional implementation and program evaluation, educators can take deliberate steps to successfully formalize HSS in the clinical environment and help move away from the prevailing hidden curriculum of the clinical workplace.

TAKE-HOME POINTS

1. Educators should begin by leveraging resources and clinical environments that are readily available and will involve the least amount of resistance.
2. Educators should take a systematic approach to implementing HSS content into CEs.
3. Educators should develop a plan for learner assessment and program evaluation that is appropriate for the CLE.

QUESTIONS FOR FURTHER THOUGHT

1. Before embarking on this journey, why is it essential that educators consider the continuum of training?
2. What are examples of tools and resources educators can use to assist with implementing HSS training in the CLE?
3. What are key considerations educators should address in advance when planning for the successful implementation of HSS training in the clinical environment for medical students?

VIGNETTE

The clerkship program directors at your medical school are invited to a faculty meeting to discuss curricular changes and innovation in undergraduate medical education (UME). In the meeting, the medical school dean asks that all clerkship directors consider how best to teach health systems science (HSS) in their UME clinical experiences (CEs). As the medicine clerkship director, you start thinking of whether you will need to create a-half-day-per week experience discussing HSS topics in the medicine clerkship. Your surgical colleague turns to you and asks for your help, saying, "It's easy to do this in medicine, but what can we do in surgery?" You decide to work with her to determine what HSS elements are best taught in the context of CEs.

Thought Questions

1. What are immediately available opportunities within the clinical learning environment that can be used to illustrate and practice HSS domains?
2. What are common challenges in integrating HSS into the clinical experience?

ANNOTATED BIBLIOGRAPHY

Jaffe RC, Bergin CR, Loo LK, et al. Nested domains: a global conceptual model for optimizing the clinical learning environment. *Am J Med.* 2019;132(7):886-891.

In this Jaffe et al. offer a conceptual model to optimize the clinical learning and working environment that promotes more effective communication and collaboration among the stakeholders that work within it. This model may offer yet another framework to help guide the implementation of HSS in the clinical learning environment for its learners.

Melle EV. Using a logic model to assist in the planning, implementation, and evaluation of educational programs. *Acad Med.* 2016;91(10):1464.

In this Academic Medicine Last Page, Melle introduces the logic model as an approach to program planning, implementation, and evaluation. The authors introduce logic model basics through an example and share tips for successfully using and applying logic models.

Topor DR, Dickey C, Stonestreet L, Wendt J, Woolley A, Budson A. Interprofessional health care education at academic medical centers: using a SWOT analysis to develop and implement programming. *MedEdPORTAL.* 2018;14:10766.

In this MedEdPORTAL submission, Topor et al. share a workshop to teach educators how to apply a SWOT analysis for the development of training programs that incorporate interprofessional practice and education.

REFERENCES

1. Lehmann LS, Sulmasy LS, Desai S, ACP Ethics, Professionalism and Human Rights Committee. Hidden curricula, ethics, and professionalism: optimizing clinical learning environments in becoming and being a physician: a position paper of the American College of Physicians. *Ann Intern Med.* 2018;168(7):506-508.
2. Jaffe RC, Bergin CR, Loo LK, et al. Nested domains: a global conceptual model for optimizing the clinical learning environment. *Am J Med.* 2019;132(7):886-891.
3. Papanagnou D, Jaffe R, Ziring D. Highlighting a curricular need: uncertainty, COVID-19, and health systems science. *Health Sci Rep.* 2021;4(3):e363.
4. Gonzalo JD, Hammoud MM, Starr SR. Systems thinking in health care: addressing the complex dynamics of patients and health systems. In: Skochelak SE, Hammoud MM, Lomis KD, et al., eds. *AMA Medical Education Consortium: Health Systems Science.* 2nd ed. Philadelphia: Elsevier; 2021:21-36.
5. Adams NE. Bloom's taxonomy of cognitive learning objectives. *J Med Libr Assoc.* 2015;103(3):152-153.
6. Topor DR, Dickey C, Stonestreet L, Wendt J, Woolley A, Budson A. Interprofessional health care education at academic medical centers: using a SWOT analysis to develop and implement programming. *MedEdPORTAL.* 2018;14:10766.
7. Ziring D, Berg K, Mingioni N, Papanagnou D, Vaid U, Herrine S. Sidney Kimmel Medical College at Thomas Jefferson University. *Acad Med.* 2020;95(suppl 9):S444-S448.
8. Sidney Kimmel Medical College at Thomas Jefferson University. *Undergraduate Medical Education.* Available at: https://www.jefferson.edu/academics/colleges-schools-institutes/skmc/undergraduate-medical-education/curriculum.html. Accessed April 12, 2022.
9. Melle EV. Using a logic model to assist in the planning, implementation, and evaluation of educational programs. *Acad Med.* 2016;91(10):1464.
10. Balmer DF, Hall E, Fink M, Richards BF. How do medical students navigate the interplay of explicit curricula, implicit curricula, and extracurricula to learn curricular objectives? *Acad Med.* 2013;88(8):1135-1141.
11. Miller School of Medicine, University of Miami. *Office of Curriculum (Office of Medical Education).* https://med.miami.edu/en/medical-education/divisions/curriculum. Accessed April 12, 2022.
12. Miller School of Medicine, University of Miami. *Medicine as a Profession (MAP).* Available at: https://med.miami.edu/en/medical-education/divisions/curriculum/map. Accessed April 12, 2022.
13. Southern Illinois University School of Medicine. *Education and Curriculum.* Available at: https://www.siumed.edu/oec. Accessed April 12, 2022.
14. Perelman School of Medicine, University of Pennsylvania. *Measey Primary Care Pathway: Courses and Workshops.* Available at: https://www.med.upenn.edu/primarycarepathway/courses-and-workshops.html. Accessed April 12, 2022.
15. Ten Cate, O. Entrustment decisions: bringing the patient into the assessment equation. *Acad Med.* 2017;92(6):736-738.

Health Systems Science Implementation in Graduate Medical Education

Casey Olm-Shipman, Tracey L. Henry, and Dharmini Shah Pandya

LEARNING OBJECTIVES

1. Discuss the case for integrating health systems science (HSS) into graduate medical education (GME) programming and curricula.
2. Create an approach to integrate HSS into GME that considers the common challenges faculty may encounter.
3. Identify faculty development and infrastructure needs for successful implementation and sustainment of HSS in GME.
4. Explore assessment and evaluation strategies to measure the impact of HSS programming and curricula on learners, teachers, and patient health outcomes.

CHAPTER OUTLINE

Chapter Summary, 66
Making the Case for Health Systems Science in Graduate Medical Education, 66
  Unique Challenges to Health Systems Science Development and Implementation in the Context of Graduate Medical Education Training, 66
  Return-on-Investment Opportunities for HSS within GME, 67
  Alignment With GME Program Credentialing Requirements, 67
  Developing GME Trainees as Change Agents, 67
  Alignment with Health System Organizational Goals, 68
  Alignment with Institutional Mission to Support Learning Across the Medical Education Continuum, 68
  Summary of Challenges and Barriers for Implementation of Health Systems Science in Graduate Medical Education and Strategies to Overcome Them, 68
Faculty Development and Creating Sustainable Infrastructure, 68
  Creating Buy-in and Value with Faculty, 68

  Identifying Faculty and Infrastructural Resource Needs, 69
  Identifying Educational and Development Opportunities, 70
  Challenges and Barriers, 72
  Strategies and Approaches for Faculty Development, 72
Approach to Integration of Health Systems Science, 72
  Kern's Six-Step Approach to Curriculum Development and Application, 74
  The Accreditation Council for GME Clinical Learning Environment Review Framework, 79
  Evaluation of Individual Learners Using the Accreditation Council for Graduate Medical Education Core Competencies Framework, 80
  Evaluation of Health Systems Science Educators, 82
  Evaluation of the Impact of Health Systems Science Programming on Patient Health Outcomes, 82
Take-Home Points, 83
Questions for Further Thought, 83

CHAPTER SUMMARY

The objective of this chapter is to apply knowledge and skills in the development and integration of a health systems science (HSS) curriculum in the clinical learning environment within graduate medical education (GME). We focus on the challenges, barriers, and successes in the development, integration, and evaluation of HSS into curricula for residents and fellows. We begin the discussion in the chapter with outlining the argument for HSS in GME followed by key principles to be considered, including the approach to integration, faculty development, and assessment and evaluation strategies. We conclude the discussion with case vignettes and concrete discussion points that can be used in the development and integration of HSS at the program and institutional GME levels.

MAKING THE CASE FOR HEALTH SYSTEMS SCIENCE IN GRADUATE MEDICAL EDUCATION

Integrating HSS into GME is essential for training doctors who are better prepared to deliver exceptional patient care in increasingly complex health systems. Although few would debate the urgent need for innovative training pathways that deliver on the Quadruple Aim to reduce costs, improve population health, better the patient experience, and increase health care team well-being,[1] successful development and implementation of HSS programming in the GME environment remains uniquely challenging. Because of a relative lack of expert-driven and evidence-based guidelines to inform best practices, devising a pathway forward can be a daunting task for those who work in GME.

Unique Challenges to HSS Development and Implementation in the Context of GME Training

Despite increasing agreement that HSS domains are critical to teaching and assessment throughout the continuum of undergraduate medical education (UME) to GME, there are multiple barriers and challenges. Emphasis on HSS education is highlighted in the Accreditation Council for Graduate Medical Education (ACGME) Milestones 2.0 and Clinical Learning Environment Review (CLER) recommendations, which have led to significant changes in the evaluation of trainees. However, HSS content is not uniformly executed because of the breadth of information, inconsistent teaching methods, and a lack of evidence that HSS curricula improves education or population outcomes.

One of the most distinct barriers to HSS programming commonly encountered by educators within the GME environment are regulations restricting residents to an 80-hour work week. GME trainees serve on the front lines of clinical operations and care delivery. Given the intensity of clinical demands, GME trainees and faculty are vulnerable to running on "negative time" when engaging in new educational programming. Unlike medical students, whose primary role is as a learner on the health care team, residents and fellows are both learners and major parts of the physician workforce in their hospitals and clinics. As such, many ACGME-affiliated hospitals and clinics could not continue clinical operations without GME trainees. Compared with medical students, time for dedicated educational programming is significantly more compressed. Additionally, because formal HSS education has been historically underresourced within the culture of GME training, it is particularly vulnerable to deprioritization by overly burdened trainees, faculty, and health care system leaders, who may perceive learning about HSS to be non–value-added "extra work" without immediate benefit. The lack of infrastructure and faculty development pathways to support sustainable HSS programming further exacerbates this issue.

An additional layer of complexity to implementation of HSS within the GME environment is the need to prioritize content that teaches the core clinical knowledge and skills necessary to pass specialty board examinations. Unlike in UME, in which the National Board of Medical Examiners (NBME) offers a dedicated HSS evaluation to assess medical student knowledge, specialty certification board examinations have traditionally emphasized the application of medical knowledge to diagnose and manage patients with disease conditions.[2] Additionally, how HSS competencies are tested meaningfully and with validity has not been established. Hence, the incentive to learn and teach HSS for the purpose of passing board examinations is currently limited.

Another significant factor impacting the ability to integrate HSS within GME is the diametrically centralized–decentralized structure of GME within institutions in which a multitude of specialty training programs may exist. Whereas programs under one institutional umbrella may share many overarching standards, each resident and fellowship specialty program within a single institution is beholden to the clinical workflows and educational infrastructure of their respective academic departments and clinical service lines. Residency programs and their trainees are embedded within diverse specialties caring for different patient populations with heterogeneous disease conditions. As such, HSS experiences are highly contextualized within specialty-based GME clinical learning environments, leading to the creation of stand-alone programs as opposed to those that integrate with the clinical learning environment as part of the routine approach to care delivery. Even within a single institution, there is considerable variation between residency training programs regarding the existence, quality, and integration of HSS within each program's curriculum. Variation is likely further compounded when comparing training programs across institutions. It is therefore not surprising that implementation of centralized HSS programming that is accessible, relevant, and value-added to GME trainees across specialties, both within and between institutions, poses considerable hurdles.

Return-on-Investment Opportunities for HSS Within GME

Given these distinct challenges within the GME clinical learning environment, the development and integration of effective and sustainable HSS programming requires an investment of resources, sponsorship, and stakeholder buy-in. Securing these resources is vital to the success of these programs as well as the continued engagement of clinical educators and trainees who lead, teach, and learn within them. Without adequate resources, HSS programming may rely on the underrecognized and undervalued efforts of a few select individuals. Rarely are such approaches sustainable or scalable, and even worse, this approach may result in clinician educator burnout as well as inequitable taxation of faculty time without clear career advancement benefit (e.g., academic promotion) for those who lead and contribute to HSS programs.

In making the return-on-investment case for HSS within the GME environment, we find it helpful to identify where shared vested interests between stakeholders exist and then leverage win–win opportunities. This usually entails alignment of HSS in GME with at least one of several key organizational priorities and is vital to securing institutional resources for HSS program development, implementation, and sustainability. There are four, major organizational priorities common to many academic institutions, which effective HSS programming has the potential to significantly impact:

- Residency and fellowship program credentialing, which depends on adherence to CLER recommendations and trainees meeting ACGME Milestones
- Developing front-line clinicians as effective change agents to foster high-reliability organizations

- Achieving health system organizational goals, particularly those pertaining to value-based care, health equity, and patient outcomes
- Supporting institutional mission to promote learning across the medical education continuum inclusive of medical students, GME trainees, and faculty

Alignment With GME Program Credentialing Requirements

Because GME trainees are essential to the workforce in academic medicine, health care system leadership and residency program directors must prioritize credentialing of ACGME programs to maintain the clinical operations of hospitals and clinics. As part of program credentialing, it is mandatory that ACGME training programs adhere to CLER recommendations and ACGME Milestones. Embedded within these recommendations and milestones are several core domains encompassed by HSS, including patient safety, health care quality, care transitions, well-being, and professionalism. As HSS educators, if we can build programs that support credentialing and facilitate adherence to CLER and ACGME requirements, this is a significant win for multiple stakeholders. Furthermore, if educators can create opportunities for collaboration and sharing of resources through the development of HSS programs, this also reduces workload redundancy for faculty who may be teaching in decentralized GME siloes across the institution (which in turn may prove helpful in preventing burnout).

Developing GME Trainees as Change Agents

Graduate medical education trainees are uniquely positioned to operate as effective change agents because they are the physicians on the front lines of care delivery in the academic medical center. They are arguably the most experienced in confronting, navigating, and solving systems-based practice issues that emerge in the process of delivering patient care. As the clinicians who are often most knowledgeable of the nuances of clinical operations pertaining to clinics, wards, and operating rooms, they may be the most attuned to gaps, deficiencies, and opportunities for system improvement. Additionally, as the front-line care team members, they are major stakeholders in improvement efforts because these efforts may directly impact their daily practice. As such, when trainees are engaged as change agents, they can significantly enhance care delivery, introducing new and creative change ideas that are meaningful to local systems. As front-line drivers of change, they also directly experience the benefits of their improvement efforts, which can bolster satisfaction and perpetuate a vested interest in bettering the systems in which they work.[3]

Alignment With Health System Organizational Goals

In a rapidly evolving health care landscape in which costly diagnostic and therapeutic advances have often failed to translate to improved patient outcomes at the population health level, implementation of successful value-based care is of critical importance.[4] In the United States, quality measurement has expanded exponentially, with the goal of improving outcomes, preventing harm, and improving the patient experience. Additionally, quality measures are used to identify gaps in practice and unwarranted variation that contributes to health inequities. Since the Patient Protection and Affordable Care Act became law in 2010, there has been an active shift from fee-for-service to value-based care models.[5,6] As a result, quality measures tracked by health care organizations are increasingly tied to publicly reported benchmarking programs, national credentialing standards, and financial reimbursement. It has therefore become a financial imperative for health care organizations and care teams to prioritize quality, resulting in significant administrative expenditure.[7,8] In the academic medical center, the ability of trainees to successfully engage in systems-based care and apply HSS principles to daily clinical practice has the potential to greatly affect clinical outcomes and organizational performance measures.[9] When up to 6% of hospital reimbursement is at risk through federally mandated Centers for Medicare & Medicaid Services (CMS) pay-for-performance programs, hospital administrations and medical educators cannot afford to neglect HSS in the GME clinical learning environment.[10–12]

Alignment With Institutional Mission to Support Learning Across the Medical Education Continuum

For an academic medical center, education of medical students, residents, fellows, and faculty across the continuum is central to mission. Just as faculty must teach and support residents and fellows in the clinical learning environment, so must residents and fellows teach and support medical students during their clinical clerkship years. Medical schools in the United States are increasingly prioritizing HSS within their formal classroom curriculums. However, whether and how medical student HSS learning translates to the clinical learning environment once students enter clinical clerkships is largely uncharted territory. Because residents and fellows provide significant modeling and teaching to medical students during their clerkships, if medical students are to learn how to apply HSS principles at the bedside, then residents and fellows must have the knowledge and skills to teach them. Likewise, faculty must also be competent in HSS if they are to educate both UME and GME learners in practice. To create synergy and harmonization between the HSS-related core competencies valued by both UME and GME, accessible HSS training must be available to all learners across the medical education continuum.

Summary of Challenges and Barriers for Implementation of Health Systems Science in Graduate Medical Education and Strategies to Overcome Them

- Competing demands of clinical and didactic responsibilities, limited faculty development support, siloing of HSS programming, and lack of prioritization of HSS within the GME environment all represent significant barriers to successful integration and sustainment of HSS initiatives.
- The key to overcoming these barriers is leveraging alignment with institutional and organizational goals. By developing GME trainees as effective change agents and aligning HSS initiatives with GME credentialing requirements, organizational goals, and institutional educational mission across the learning continuum, HSS leaders may garner institutional support and buy-in necessary for successful program development and implementation.

FACULTY DEVELOPMENT AND CREATING SUSTAINABLE INFRASTRUCTURE

Creating Buy-in and Value With Faculty

Undoubtedly, the most important part of any new curriculum is the faculty. For any new curriculum, including HSS curriculum, to be effective, it must be accepted by faculty and deemed educationally valid.[13] Ideally, faculty are made active participants early in the development of the new curriculum.[14] In considering which faculty to engage, we suggest prioritizing the motivated and energetic faculty who may have reached out to participate or who have previously worked in HSS-related areas. We also recommend proactively reaching out to junior faculty who are building up their knowledge or skill sets in HSS content areas.

Fetters et al.[15] notes that the stages of developing a new curriculum can be matched to stages of faculty development (Fig. 5.1). They use the three innovator categories—early adopter, early majority, and late majority—to describe the stages of faculty development, which type of faculty should be engaged at each stage, and the type of faculty development needed. Early adopters are the faculty who have been involved in various levels of HSS curriculum either as a

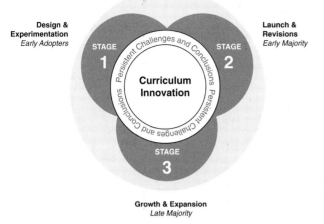

Design &
Experimentation
Early Adopters

STAGE 1

Persistent Challenges and Conclusions

Curriculum Innovation

Launch & Revisions
Early Majority

STAGE 2

Persistent Challenges and Conclusions

STAGE 3

Growth & Expansion
Late Majority

Fig. 5.1 Stages of blended learning faculty development. (Reprinted with permission from Fetters ML, Duby TG. Faculty development: a stage model matched to blended learning maturation. *JALN.* 2011;15(1):77-86.)

student or resident; involved through prior experiences or job roles; or have prior curriculum design experiences in HSS related topics such as quality improvement, patient safety, advocacy, or policy. They have the basic level of curriculum design and teaching experience from which to build on and can even suggest innovative methods of teaching. These faculty members have intrinsic buy-in; they understand both the assignment and what needs to be changed. Faculty development should be tailored for each early adopter based on their background in HSS or their planned contribution. For example, a faculty member who has worked in health care policy for 20 years but is new to academic medicine may need more faculty development in curricular design and teaching methods, and another faculty member who has developed several successful courses but is new to HSS will require knowledge and content acquisition. Faculty who are early adopters should be chosen, supported (including with a full-time equivalent [FTE] salary and stipends for curricular support), and recognized by their departments to ensure sustainability of the new HSS curriculum.[15]

In the early majority stage, the HSS curriculum has started to take shape. The curriculum has been designed, and the early adopter faculty appear to be thriving. This is when we add additional faculty who were initially hesitant to participate but now are intrigued and want to be involved. At this stage, faculty still require tailored faculty development, which can be incorporated into ongoing faculty development efforts. Examples of tailored faculty development include workshops, seminars, or didactics on whichever skill set the faculty member is lacking, such as curriculum development in HSS, optional ways to teach HSS (workshops, flipped classrooms, bedside, experiential), and how to evaluate learners in HSS curricula.

In the late majority stage, we suggest addressing the faculty who did not see value in the new HSS curriculum initially and even now view it with some skepticism. They need to see the curriculum achieve some wins before participating. The goal is to minimize the concerns regarding interjecting more content in an already limited amount of academic curricular space and time. One strategy already discussed is to create buy-in and obtain approval and co-operation from both institutional GME offices and individual program directors. Top-down approval and buy-in will mitigate barriers in obtaining funding for implementation, programmatic support, FTE for instructors, and dedicated time for faculty development. By investing in FTE so that faculty can participate in the faculty development process, including curriculum planning and assessment, we instill faculty ownership of the curriculum. Communicating the need for change repeatedly through email, departmental newsletters, and meetings will keep the momentum going and the sense of urgency intriguing to many, thereby creating further buy-in.[16] The specific faculty development strategy for the late majority is to engage them in maintaining the HSS curriculum. These late adopters can pinch hit or begin to fill in the spaces where faculty who are early or majority adopters may have grown fatigued. At this stage, faculty development should include incentives for curriculum innovation, resources, and support for late adopters to review what work has been done and ways to continue to push the HSS curriculum forward.

Identifying Faculty and Infrastructural Resource Needs

Those working to implement an HSS curriculum in GME should identify resources to support the inclusion of other expert teachers and prioritize efforts to engage these teachers. Obtaining support begins with engaging key stakeholders spanning from the medical school deans, health care system leaders, and community leaders along with highlighting shared missions and their alignment with an HSS curriculum. Engaged leaders can champion the curriculum, identify available resources and stakeholders, and identify other groups working on similar goals.

In identifying faculty development needs, we recommend first conducting an assessment to determine (1) faculty needs, knowledge, interest, and availability to teach the HSS curricula; (2) ways the HSS curriculum can be incorporated within the current infrastructure or what changes need to be made to the current infrastructure; and, (3) a climate survey to assess the sentiments of faculty and staff toward implementing a new HSS curricula. In the needs assessment, faculty can rate their knowledge and skills specific to HSS curricula and identify gaps in knowledge and skills. The needs assessment also identifies gaps in the current professional faculty development training as it relates to HSS. As a final point, the needs assessment is key to reassuring program faculty and staff that implementation will not be haphazard but a well-thought-out effort. The climate survey should assess the aforementioned buy-in, assist in driving cultural change, and identify priority areas of concerns to address. The climate change survey should also elucidate the strengths, weaknesses, opportunities, and threats in regard to faculty engagement for the HSS curriculum.

In evaluating current infrastructure needs, faculty have to consider where and when in the curriculum HSS will be implemented, how many instructors are needed, and whether there will be one instructor for all lectures or multiple instructors or guest lectures. Other infrastructure needs include dedicated programmatic administrative support, an identified HSS faculty curriculum lead (or leads) to oversee the curriculum and lead the development and implementation efforts, and budget and funding for faculty instructors and their faculty development. Additionally, as evidence of buy-in, the HSS curriculum should be highlighted by GME programs as a part of core curriculum appropriately listed on GME program websites and brochures in GME recruitment efforts. Finally, faculty have to identify instructional materials including, textbooks, podcasts, peer-reviewed journal articles, policy papers, and experiences along with organizing a well-structured coherent curriculum for the bedside or the classroom.

Identifying Educational and Development Opportunities

Typically, faculty members are not trained to teach before being hired as educators, and this is no different as it relates to the HSS curriculum. Faculty, however, teach in ways similar to how they were taught, and learn throughout career and experiences, and learn through faculty development programs.[17] Thus, from the needs assessment, curriculum designers are able to create and tailor educational and faculty development opportunities for the specific GME program. This includes the chance to "teach the teachers" by developing the faculty's knowledge and skills in implementing the HSS curriculum via a comprehensive faculty development program. Teaching the teachers can come in various forms, via outsourcing faculty development by sending a faculty member (or members) to HSS-related curriculum training programs, programs related to various HSS content areas, curriculum development programs or workshops, or "learning how to be better teachers training programs." A barrier to implementing HSS is the newness of the field and the fact that most faculty were not formally trained in HSS. Although they may have learned much of the content on the fly as their careers have progressed, they are unclear how to teach it. Thus, these faculty development opportunities uniquely empower faculty to not only desire to teach and embrace HSS into their GME programs but also make them into better teachers and clinicians. Faculty development activities ensure the integrity of the HSS curriculum and the desired quality of instruction after implementation.[18]

After faculty needs have been established (Table 5.1), curriculum designers should identify the focus, learning

TABLE 5.1   General Needs Assessment for Faculty: Aimed at Teaching Ability

GME Faculty Needs Assessment for Health Systems Science Curriculum

Are you aware of HSS? (Y/N)	
Have you ever developed a curriculum before? (Y/N)	
I see value in integrating HSS into our current curriculum (select one):	Strongly agree, Agree, Neutral, Disagree, Strongly disagree
Please list any prior experiential, bedside teaching, or experiences related to HSS. (Please comment.)	

TABLE 5.1	General Needs Assessment for Faculty: Aimed at Teaching Ability—cont'd			
Have you ever taught in an HSS curricula before? (Y/N)				
	Which HSS domains have you previously taught?	Please rate knowledge level in each HSS core domain (select one): Expert, Above average knowledge, Average knowledge, Minimal knowledge, No knowledge	Please rate confidence level in teaching HSS curricula in each core domain: Very confident, Confident, Neutral, Somewhat confident, Not confident	Please rate ability to evaluate GME learners in HSS by domain: Expert, Above average knowledge or skills, Average knowledge or skills, Minimal knowledge or skills, No knowledge or skills
Health Systems Science Core Domains				
Patient, family, and community				
Health care policy and economics				
Population, public, and structural and social determinants of health				
Value in health care				
Clinical informatics and health technology				
Teaming				
Leadership				
Systems thinking				
Ethics and legal				
Change agency, management, and advocacy				
Health system improvement				
Health care structure and process				
Feedback, comments, and concerns				

GME, Graduate medical education; HSS, health systems science.

goals, and frequency and type of training. For faculty who are aiming to become HSS content experts or want to sharpen their current HSS content knowledge, those implementing an HSS curriculum should select from one of the twelve **HSS core domains**. Of note, in our approach to faculty development, we include training faculty to not only teach learners in the traditional classroom format but also how to integrate teaching and evaluation of learners using HSS at the bedside or experientially. Faculty and professional development training can take the form of lectures, 1- to 2-hour workshops, seminars, or courses.[19] When faculty become proficient in HSS knowledge content, curriculum building, and teaching methods, providing one-on-one mentoring of newly identified faculty HSS teachers is a key part of infrastructure building for sustainability.[14]

If there is a dearth of available faculty to teach in a new HSS curriculum, whether it is from a lack of interest, expertise, or availability, faculty from other departments, adjacent schools of public health, or other related fields can be recruited. In fact, having content experts who have actually worked in the related HSS content-related fields and have real-world experience can show how HSS is used in practice. Using community and institutional experts to teach and set standards in relevant HSS domains for faculty is an important pillar to curricular efforts.

Collaborative efforts across health profession disciplines are required to consistently integrate newly learned concepts into practice by faculty, improve outcomes, and role model new competencies to trainees and colleagues.

Another area of opportunity for infrastructure building is for faculty to reach out to other programs that have successfully built HSS into their GME programs for best practices and pitfalls to avoid. More established HSS program leaders can also mentor programs in the beginning stages of implementation. Evaluations from learners will help identify areas for further improvement, including faculty development needs. Similarly judicious is evaluating the effectiveness of a program at the end of each academic year by way of pre-identified metrics for success and making curricular enhancements as needed to meet learner needs.

Challenges and Barriers

Well-cited barriers to curriculum development, implementation, and faculty development include:[20]
- Lack of buy-in along with misconceptions about perceived value and relevance of the new curriculum.
- Lack of motivation and resistance to change.
- Lack of funding for curriculum, FTE, or faculty release time to participate in faculty development activities.
- Lack of time for, access to, and awareness of the new curriculum content.

Strategies and Approaches for Faculty Development
- Planning faculty development in the HSS curriculum begins with identifying the needs of the faculty members involved.
- To identify faculty development and infrastructure needs, it is best to begin with a needs assessment and climate survey.
- Goals of faculty development include:
  - Becoming HSS content leaders.
  - Learning curriculum development.
  - Learning HSS teaching methods.
  - Determining how to integrate HSS in different teaching settings.
  - Building confidence in teaching HSS.
  - Developing skills to evaluate GME learners in HSS.
- Tailor faculty development and strategic planning to the results of the needs assessment and climate survey.
- Financial and programmatic support is prudent.
- Ongoing assessment and monitoring of the curriculum and the flexibility to pivot is key.

APPROACH TO INTEGRATION OF HEALTH SYSTEMS SCIENCE

In this section, we discuss best practices and principles for an approach to HSS integration that addresses barriers and challenges that are unique to the GME infrastructure. HSS is unparalleled in GME in that it is both a framework for critical systems thinking, and its individual parts such as high-value care, quality improvement, and health policy can be considered their own lone-standing curricula. New generations of educators who create curricula have to adapt to a rapidly changing practice landscape. They must be equipped to build curricula that not only emphasizes basic and clinical sciences but also must integrate foundational skills that allow learners to innovate within their health care environment and deliver holistic patient care. In addition, it is important to keep in mind, when approaching evaluation of the GME trainee in domains encompassed by HSS, that faculty and residency program directors charged with assessing and evaluating GME trainee performance may themselves have little formal education pertaining to HSS concepts and application in practice. If our educators performing the assessments are not well-versed in HSS and lack a clearly defined, specific, and standardized rubric to guide evaluation, the effectiveness and validity of learner assessments are difficult to know.

Building curricula and assessment can be done through the lens of HSS to achieve a sustainable practice environment through a systematic approach which is linked to health care needs.[21] This can be done by using the widely adopted "six-step approach" by Kern as described in Chapter 1. Here we discuss the GME application of the "six-step approach," which provides a pragmatic framework that is widely applicable but can be tailored to institutional culture and values. The goal of HSS curricula is to provide opportunities for trainees and faculty to become **change agents**, develop growth mindset skills, and have a meaningful contribution to system changes.

Kern's approach to curriculum can be utilized to integrate HSS concepts in a simple, logical, and practical way so that sustainable and flexible curricular changes can occur.

The assumptions of this methodology include all educational programs have aims and goals; medical educators have a professional and ethical obligation to meet the needs of their learners, patients, and society; and medical educators should be held accountable for the outcomes of their interventions.[22] A foundational pillar of any endeavor that incorporates integration of HSS curricula in GME is recognition that curricula must expand beyond the widely accepted singular didactic approach to curricula, and efforts must extend into the learning practice environment.[21]

Refer to Box 5.1 for a stepwise application of Kern's six steps to high-value care curriculum with an HSS lens to GME.

BOX 5.1　High-Value Care Curriculum Implementation Through the HHS Lens: Kern's Six-Step Application to GME

Step 1: Problem Identification
Traditional approach: Teaching high-value care (HVC) is a basic requirement in GME with ACGME Milestones because this drives diagnostic reasoning and skills.

Ideal approach: Health care costs in the United States are increasing at an unsustainable rate. Approximately 30% of health care costs are wasted care, care that is potentially avoidable and would not negatively affect the quality of care if eliminated. There is growing concern that medical expenditures are contributing significantly to the federal deficit and the United States' weakening economy. Wasted care includes overuse and misuse of diagnostic testing, avoidable hospitalization and rehospitalization, and overuse of ED services. GME provides an opportunity to shape the habits of future physicians regarding cost consciousness and stewardship of resources, especially as it imprints their long-term practice behaviors.

Step 2: Targeted Needs Assessment
Assess HVC from the perspective of a learner, faculty member, and health care system.

Step 3: Goals and Objectives
At the completion of residency, internal medicine residents will be able to provide care that meets the Quadruple Aim: better care for individual patients, better health for populations, better provider satisfaction, and lower health costs.
- PGY1: Learners will be able to define value, quality, as defined by the Quadruple Aim.
- PGY1/2/3: Learners will be able to discuss value and cost during rounds and patient encounters in the context of understanding the benefits, harms, and relative costs of the interventions that are being considered.
- PGY2/3: Learners will be able to customize a care plan with each patient that incorporates the patient's values and addresses patient and family concerns.

- PGY2/3: Learners will be able to identify patterns of social determinants of health and inequity in access to health care on their patient panels.
- PGY3: Learners discuss one way the curriculum has helped them learn about how systems and HVC affects the health of community members.

Step 4: Educational Strategies
Formal curricula: sequential curricula based on training year.
- PGY1: Formal dedicated didactics, ACP's HVC modules; define the Quadruple Aim definition of value.
- PGY1/2/3: Incorporate into their clinical reasoning didactics different approaches to workup and treatment based on cost, access, and utility.

Informal: Have attendings specifically address value when ordering tests and treatments for patients while caring for patients in clinic or the wards.

Hidden: Have the faculty role model having a cost of care conversation with patients when addressing non–value-added diagnostic tests that were requested by the family or patient.

Experiential: Work with the utilization review department to uncover the costs to the patients and health care system. Identify system-level opportunities to improve outcomes, minimize harms, and reduce health care waste and carry out a quality improvement project related to this opportunity.

Step 5: Implementation
Dedicated time for explicit HVC concepts during general medicine didactics.
- PGY1: Dedicated didactic series to develop common language and nomenclature. Accountability to complete modules asynchronously.
- PGY2/3: Incorporate into current didactic series and use explicit labeling of "the HVC concept" embedded into clinical reasoning series.

Continued

Have patients speak about their experience after receiving a bill post hospitalization with a reflection session.

Discussions on rounds about value, diagnostic tests, treatments, and value-added versus non–value-added services. Attendings to give explicit feedback on skills related to HVC: diagnostic test ordering practices and value conversations.

Step 6: Evaluation and Assessment
Learner skills evaluation: Use Milestone 2.0 from the ACGME with the mapped milestones to HSS.

Curricula assessment: Incorporate into the programmatic end-of-year survey and didactic surveys.

Faculty feedback: Schedule regular interval feedback sessions about HVC and the ability to incorporate on rounds.

ACGME, Accreditation Council for Graduate Medical Education; *ACP,* American College of Physicians; *ED,* emergency department; *GME,* graduate medical education; *HSS,* health systems science; *HVC,* high-value care; *PGY,* postgraduate year.

Kern's Six-Step Approach to Curriculum Development and Application

Step 1: Identify the Problem

The first step is to start with the identification and analysis of a health care need or other problem that is to be addressed by the curriculum. Clear definition of the problem is the foundation that allows for attainable curriculum goals and objectives, which in turn helps to focus the curriculum's educational and evaluation strategies. The goal is to create an evidence-based argument for the need to create a new curriculum, which must extend beyond traditional learner-centric needs.[21]

Completing this first step requires awareness of existing program competencies, but HSS curricula creators must elevate programs by using **systems thinking** to go beyond the individual needs of trainees, physicians, and other health care professionals. Content creators for curricula must address the epidemiology and determinants of health that affect patient outcomes at the societal level. There are several resources that can be helpful in garnering a compelling evidence base to create a burning platform for HSS curriculum development. At the national level, these include reports referenced by the National Academies of Sciences, Engineering, and Medicine on the various domains within HSS; the curriculum inventory maintained by the Association of American Medical Colleges; and MedEdPORTAL's Diversity, Inclusion, and Health Equity collection.[21]

Clear problem identification leads to an expanded competency expectation to include skills that health professionals should possess to address the identified gaps in health systems and population health.[21]

Step 2: Needs Assessment

The second step is to perform a thorough needs assessment to ensure the comprehensive development of a curricular framework that integrates the large variety of topics that can

be addressed in an HSS curriculum. The difference between how the problem is currently being addressed and how it should ideally be addressed is the general needs assessment. The aim of the needs assessment is to ensure an educational intervention is directed at the appropriate stakeholder needs and will solve a health care problem with an evidence-based approach. With the problem statement in mind, medical educators should identify the most important and applicable content necessary for GME curricula.[21]

Because HSS content addresses health care system gaps, a full scope of current curricular needs and gaps is imperative. Unlike the problem statement, an approach to the needs assessment emphasizes the baseline viewpoints, attitudes, and behaviors of individual learners, faculty, and the health system at large.[21] Multiple methods should be used to approach an individual party's needs assessment. Modalities can include informal discussions with stakeholders, formal interviews, focus group discussions, anonymous questionnaires or surveys, direct observation of skills, examinations, audits of current performance, or strategic planning sessions with content leaders.[22]

Our approach to the program's needs assessment includes elements of a gap analysis and needs assessment from the level of a learner, faculty, and health system (Tables 5.2 and 5.3). The outline of an HSS needs assessment includes multiple domains and considerations: a traditional approach to the specified topics, an HSS approach to topics, current state of content, who is teaching the topic, barriers to teaching the topic, key stakeholders, and next steps that can be clearly delineated. A gap analysis and needs assessment will help inform the goals and objectives, assessment tools, and implementation strategies.

Step 3: Learning Goals and Objectives

The third step requires a refined goal statement and specific, measurable learning objectives. The goal statement generally describes the content and the purpose of the curriculum. The learning objectives clearly communicate the

TABLE 5.2 High-Value Care Curricula Gap Analysis (Pre-implementation Phase, Step 2 of Kern's Six Steps)[a]

Gap Analysis: HSS curricula considerations when designing a needs assessment	Current Assessment in the context of HVC curricula creation
What topics should be included? Use ACGME requirements; health care needs; and learner, faculty, or health system needs assessment.	Quadruple Aim Definition of value Gaps in care in our community Health policy related to HVC Documentation practices
Does this topic exist in our explicit (formal) curriculum? If so, where, and who is teaching?	A loose adaptation of the ACP's HVC curriculum has been implemented as required modules during the PGY1 year, kept track of by the residency administrators. Otherwise not reiterated during the mainstream didactic series.
Does this exist in our implicit (informal) curriculum (e.g., clinical teaching)? If so, where, and who is teaching?	No adaptation of the language in the clinical learning environment, and faculty are unfamiliar with the HVC terminology.
Are there system or culture barriers (hidden curriculum) to HVC on this topic that need to be addressed?	Multiple barriers: delays in getting outside hospital records, and certain types of testing can lead to overordering of high-end testing that is culturally propagated; general culture of using order sets leading to a wide net of ordering tests and concern around legal liability if something is "missed."
Are there existing experiential curricula for HVC?	No existing platforms.
Who are your key stakeholders?	Direct stakeholders: GME trainees, clinical medical students, faculty. High level: nursing departments, ancillary (labs, radiology), C-suite utilization review, quality improvement leaders, informatics department.
What are your explicit next steps?	Create needs assessment based on my gap analysis. Distribute to both direct and high-level stakeholders.

[a]Each question could also be adapted to the individual components of the curricula given that high-value care (HVC) is a large topic. For example, ask these same questions when investigating documentation practices, health policy, and community resources.
ACGME, Accreditation Council for Graduate Medical Education; ACP, American College of Physicians; GME, graduate medical education; HSS, health systems science; HVC, high-value care; PGY, postgraduate year.
(Adapted and used with permission from Agrwal N, Hedges M, Starr S. Mayo Clinic Alix School of Medicine. Adaptation of the "Gap Analysis Instrument.")
Audience: Aimed at trainees, faculty, program leaders, and health system leaders.

specific knowledge and skills learners will achieve, and objectives then form the basis of learner assessment and curriculum evaluation. The Kern approach for objectives advises using the question, "Who will do how much of what by when?" to facilitate writing a specific measurable learning objective.[19] Importantly because HSS goals arise from system-level gaps, this third step requires a backwards approach to identify what learner competencies are needed to help address these gaps, which will lead to specified objectives. This specifically challenges learner-centric educational models that only focus on trainee goals, and highlights learner proficiencies needed to explicitly connect to systems and community needs.[21] This approach features HSS competency core domain goals, which are inclusive of team skills, change agency, advocacy, leadership, and systems thinking. This will be encompassed and described in the context of the goals and objectives. The ultimate goal of the integration of HSS curricula is to allow GME trainees to mold their professional identity so that it is inclusive of being a systems citizen and lifelong innovator.

TABLE 5.3   Needs Assessment Example After Gap Analysis for High-Value Care Creation (Step 2 of Kern's Six Steps)

Target Audience	HSS Domain for HVC	Assessment Question
Faculty, Learner, and Institutional Leaders	Systems thinking	Are you aware of the levels of the health care system? Are you able to identify opportunities to increase value for the health system and your individual patients?
	HVC shared language or baseline understanding	What is value to you? What is a generally accepted concept of value as defined by the Quadruple Aim? Does our system adapt this definition?
	Health equity	How does HVC contribute to learning about equitable care or health equity?
		How does the institution identify gaps in quality (safe, timely, effective, efficient, equitable, patient-centered)?
		What health disparities are apparent in the community we practice in?
		What are the most common social determinants of health in our community?
	Cultural humility	What cultures are most common in our community? How can this impact their health behaviors?
	Cross-cultural communication	What is the best way to engage patients in our community in shared decision-making? What is the best way to develop a partnership with our patients and families?
	Health policy and advocacy	Health policy relevant to HVC that is affecting our individual patients?
		Health policy relevant to HVC that is affecting our institution?
	Billing and coding	How does coding and documentation contribute to HVC?
		How does our documentation contribute to the financial wellness of the institution?
		What are the most common health insurances and payment barriers for our patients?
Physicians, Faculty, and Learners	Application of HVC	What do you feel your individual patient's relationship with evidence-based medicine and shared decision-making is? Do you engage in shared decision-making?
		Look at your patient panel in your clinic. What are some themes in your clinic that come across when thinking about HVC and population health? What quality improvement projects are happening in your program? Can you think of times when you've had to advocate for a patient's needs when ordering diagnostic testing?
Faculty, Learners, and Patients	Patient-centered practices	Do you consider how much a test or treatment will cost before ordering it?
		Do you screen for the patient cost when ordering tests or treatments?
		Do you discuss the cost and value of treatments with your patients or families?
		Do you discuss cost and value as a team?
	Assessment	Faculty: Do you believe that you have the skills to assess learners' ability to practice HVC and diagnostic decision-making and counsel patients on HVC decision-making?
		Learners: Do you believe you can give feedback and contribute to the health system about HVC practices?
		Patients: Is there an avenue that exists to give feedback to the system and providers about diagnostic testing, patient experience, shared decision-making, and indications for testing?

HSS, Health systems science; *HVC,* high-value care.

Step 4: Organizational and Educational Strategies

The fourth step emphasizes the educational methods that will be used to deliver the content of the curriculum. The choice of educational methods is critical in HSS because the method directly addresses a significant barrier, which will help shape attitudes toward systems-minded thinking.[21]

HSS widens the scope of care delivery from learners by combining basic sciences and clinical sciences, and analyzing the impact of their care. Ideally, there should be multiple areas of overlap between HSS principles in the clinical context. The general approach to curricula creation includes introduction to skills by didactic presentations, demonstrations, discussions, and an opportunity to practice skills, an opportunity to reflect on performance, and feedback on performance. This cycle is repeated until mastery is achieved. Curricula must take place in a safe and supportive learning environment.[19] Formal didactic curricula can be constrained by nomenclature without focusing on clear application, but use of formal curricula terminology must be emphasized to allow for cultivation of HSS systems-minded thinking. Embedding experiential learning allows for an in-depth dive into curricular innovation, opportunity to apply concepts from formal curricula, and development of systems-minded attitudes.

Formal curricula, also synonymous with classroom-based learning or for GME outside a patient encounter, addresses cognitive objectives such as learning nomenclature, lectures, small group discussions, and problem-solving exercises.[19] Formal curricula goals include building a shared understanding of HSS domain concepts. For example, high-value care (HVC) curricula target the high prevalence of poor knowledge of cost, benefits, and harms in care delivery. Traditionally, HVC would be discussed at large in a didactic, but then the ability to apply concepts were not accepted or reinforced in the clinical arena.

In 2012, multiple national societies championed HVC tactics through the choosing Wisely campaign and a series called "Things We Do For No Reason," which caught traction among learners and faculty across UME and GME spaces.[23,24] This created national attention and space to improve health care delivery through discussion, and encouraged learners and practicing attendings to question why they are doing what they are doing. HSS-scoped curricula not only allows for improving HVC knowledge deficits but also empowers all levels of care providers to engage in value discussions that include sensitive topics such as overuse and waste. The goal of any HVC curricula is to spur conversation about what is appropriate and necessary treatment. A shared understanding of key HSS concepts creates a common language for discussing these topics, which can be addressed through formal curricula, but this cannot be the only approach.[25]

Integration of HSS into the larger formal curricular design allows for opportunity to complement and embed HSS concepts without a siloed curriculum that only emphasizes HSS nomenclature. Detailed opportunities to discuss HSS concepts through the lenses of HVC, structural and social determinants of health, health policy, and so on should be built into formal curricula structure that emphasizes clinical concepts and reasoning. For example, highlighting social and structural determinants of health concepts during a congestive heart failure management presentation is an efficient way of incorporating HSS principles during traditional didactics. Threading HSS concepts into case scenarios and existing structures allows for seamless integration and application of systems thinking in an integrative fashion. This in turn allows for seamless integration of HSS into the clinical learning environment, its application to patient care, and its impact on practice change in care delivery.[25] Explicit labeling as an HSS concept during clinical reasoning series (e.g., through an explicit colored slide or diagram indicating "HSS concept") will further integrate HSS concepts and importance into clinical reasoning and ultimately, the bedside care of patients.

Although formal curricula are important, most education at the GME level occurs in the patient care environment via informal teaching or bedside teaching.[25,26] Training programs and faculty need to role model and incorporate HSS integration into everyday clinical interactions and discussions in the scope of clinical practice is imperative. HSS nomenclature and concepts must become common language in the practice space. Shared knowledge of HSS principles throughout an institution can create a foundation for practice change and can have an impact on care delivery. Aligning educational efforts with ongoing HSS efforts within the health system provides a clear and commonly agreed on goal that can be discussed and reinforced in the clinical environment.[25]

Outside of **informal curricula**, programs may integrate explicit nonclinical opportunities for trainees to experience the patient population or health system they work in outside of a clinical setting. An example of experiential educational opportunities is community engagement curricula. These are emerging to address HSS content and to create interactive learning experiences in which trainee participation adds value to the system and the communities in which they train. The power of authentic community engagement, especially with vulnerable populations, can be transformative. Charging trainees to respond or address injustice in the communities in which they practice creates an innovative service learning opportunity within the realm of social justice and ultimately can be linked to multiple HSS domains.[27] Examples of programming include health behavior interventions in communities and schools such as peer mentoring programs for high school students interested in medicine, working with community health workers who do in-home visits and practice patient-centered advocacy, and training through social justice and philanthropic endeavors such as distribution of educational material and working to improve food security for communities.[28] Initial community engagement implementation may be superficial because significant preparation is needed to develop trusting relationships with community partners and to engage them as valued contributors to the educational process. True community-engaged medical education aligns trainee learning objectives with the community's health care needs and requires ongoing discussion and deliberation between the academic and community partners.[21,29,30]

Last, **hidden curricula** are also fundamental components of informal trainee education and represent how the majority of HSS skills are developed. Role modeling and the learner's experience in the interprofessional environment are key in forming HSS behaviors and attitudes. Addressing sensitive topics, such as hidden biases, structural and social determinants of health, health inequities, and health policy, requires methods that challenge the learners' and teachers' values, encourages personal and professional development, and provides an environment of psychological safety amenable to growth.[31,32] A common approach in UME and GME is using reflection sessions at the end of rotations or the humanities such as poetry, narratives, books, or short stories to open these conversations through gatherings called "Story Slams." A system to provide clear feedback on HSS education and clinical outcomes is an important component of hidden curricula. Providing accessible information on how individuals, teams, and the health system are performing in both discussions of value and patient care outcomes can reinforce HSS teaching opportunities and reflective practice.[25]

Many GME programs, to meet the ACGME subcompetency requirement in the ambulatory setting, are reinforcing these HSS frameworks through endeavors called "panel management." This provides trainee-specific outcome metrics related to panels to develop best practices for evidence-based guidance intervention. For example, residents are asked to review their patient-specific panels for compliance with colonoscopy screening, collective hemoglobin A1C goals, and use of risk-reduction scoring systems. This reinforces concepts from formal curricula related to population health, informal curricula through interdisciplinary care coordination, communication and documentation skill set observation, application of evidence-based guidelines, and hidden curricula from the perspective of role modeling behaviors that will shape future trainee practices. Panel management has real-time opportunity for trainee-specific feedback, intervention, and reflection at the population health level.

Alternative educational methods consideration: distinction tracks for trainees. The last curricular approach to consider for the fourth step is a distinction track for GME trainees. For individualized learner interests, a distinction track opportunity for those with specific interest in HSS can be considered. This approach can be particularly effective because the learner has often self-selected for participation.[32,33]

Initial creation of a distinction track identifies the most important and applicable content necessary for GME. Distinction tracks allow for individualized learner goals, focused on professional identity, and allow for integration of HSS seamlessly with already present curricula in the basic and clinical sciences. A track can help to create time and space without pressuring large programmatic curricular changes.

HSS rarely has one departmental home, and creating the structures to support interprofessional endeavors can be challenging.[21] Given these novel considerations, piloting the curriculum with volunteer learners and a robust evaluation plan is ideal. Facilitating qualitative feedback from all stakeholders and using a continuous quality improvement approach are critical to implementing a new curriculum within this extended educational environment, which can be manageable with engaged distinction track members.

Faculty education in HSS within a distinction track can advocate for best practices for teaching to emerge and allows for those inherently interested in HSS to contribute to the larger framework of curriculum. Distinction tracks can help inform topics for larger curricula efforts and can highlight the value of HSS topics within the individual programs landscape. Even more, tracks allow for trainees to develop into HSS leaders, to propagate and lead HSS concept learning, and to develop a cohort of peers to role model systems-minded thinking. This can elevate culture change, further integration of the HSS agenda, and lead to innate HSS leader development.

Step 5: Implementation

Step 5 of Kern's framework entails implementation by customization to an individual health system, obtaining support from across the spectrum of leaders and champions within the department, identifying existing resources, anticipating barriers, and introducing the curriculum and evaluative methods.[22]

Bridging nontraditional teachers, such as community leaders and health system financial executives, should have their expertise leveraged to expand the skill sets of learners and faculty. This avenue facilitates a sustainable clinical learning environment with perspectives of a multidisciplinary approach. During the implementation phase, emphasis must be placed on shared goal alignment and collaboration with the health care system. This provides the experiential learning opportunities required to integrate new concepts and practices into the daily work environment.[33] Implementation is a dynamic process and is crucial for successfully starting new curricular events.[19]

HSS is one pivotal piece in education reform. GME programs are designing and implementing learning activities focused on related areas because of learner needs, world events, and pressures that push for culture change within the practice of medicine. A stepwise approach to integration allows for a malleable environment in which HSS principles can drive change. Key principles for integration of HSS curricula include sustainable changes that are effective, generalizable, adaptable, and flexible. HSS does not replace but rather builds on and extends basic science and clinical frameworks already integrated into the practice environment. Throughout the stepwise approach, multiple layers of key stakeholder involvement are built in and allow for iterative evaluation of learner and community outcomes such as satisfaction, engagement, or contributions.[21] For successful curriculum implementation, the "development" stage never ends; rather, the curriculum evolves based on evaluation results, changes in resources, changes in targeted learners' needs, and changes in the material requiring mastery.[19]

Key strategies and recommendations for implementation of HSS at the GME level

- Follow a systematic approach to implementation, such as Kern's six steps, which model curricular implementation.
- Compared with traditional medical education approaches, HSS integration must address a health care need or gap, which then informs curricular content.
- HSS content should complement and expand the dimension of current didactic structures.
- A multimodal approach for implementation of HSS curricula must be considered. Strategies include addressing HSS through formal (classroom-based), informal (clinical learning), or hidden curricula (reflection, role modeling), as well as experiential learning (community or health system opportunities), and consideration of a specific HSS distinction track.
- HSS curricular efforts must emphasize professional identity formation of a systems citizen and change agency within the clinical learning environment and health system. This is key for GME learners.

Step 6: Evaluation and Feedback

Within UME, the assessment and evaluation of HSS knowledge and integration in practice has emerged as an area of increasing focus. Although assessment and evaluation of HSS learners represents a significant challenge in UME, this is amplified within GME, in which HSS assessment strategies are arguably less well developed, with comparatively little evidence base to guide clinician educators. The inherent variability that exists across each GME training specialty necessitates that HSS programming and curricula be tailored such that it is meaningful and value-added to specialty-specific GME trainees and systems of care delivery, as well as to specialty-specific heterogeneous patient populations and disease conditions. A "one-size-fits-all" approach to evaluation may therefore be less useful because general performance metrics may require significant contextualization and adaptation across specialties to be considered meaningful and relevant.

The ACGME Milestones and CLER recommendations establish the credentialing standards by which programs are assessed and provide a helpful basic guide to inform performance targets at both the individual learner and programmatic levels. It is important to keep in mind, however, that although these provide a rubric for evaluation of foundational knowledge and application in clinical practice, these measures are not necessarily developed with the degree of specificity to inform an in-depth guided assessment of an individual learner's skills and knowledge pertaining to HSS. Within UME, the NBME HSS examination is a tool that can be used for more in-depth evaluation of individual learner competency. Although standardized tests have considerable limitations in evaluating a learner's ability to apply knowledge and skills in clinical practice, they are helpful in ensuring whether foundational knowledge is taught and learned. Currently, there is no equivalent to the NBME HSS exam within GME. Within residency and fellowship programs, evaluation of the GME trainee is focused on the assessment of the following competencies: practice-based learning and improvement, patient care and procedural skills, systems-based practice; medical knowledge, interpersonal and communication skills, and professionalism. Thus, it does not provide a comprehensive assessment of all HSS competencies. In addition, HSS assessment is underrepresented (if at all) on specialty in-service and board examinations, rendering evaluation of individual HSS foundational knowledge difficult. Thus, an individual GME trainee's lack of knowledge pertaining to HSS may go undetected or not be perceived as problematic if other traditional performance metrics are satisfactorily met.

The Accreditation Council for GME Clinical Learning Environment Review Framework

As a starting point for evaluation of systems-based practice in GME, the CLER program was developed to improve engagement of resident and fellow physicians in learning to provide safe and quality care. Participating ACGME-accredited institutions undergo interval CLER site visits and receive feedback every 18 to 24 months. CLER emphasizes six domains, all overlapping with domains pertinent to HSS, including patient safety, health care quality and equity, care transitions, supervision, duty hours and fatigue management, and professionalism. Metrics within each domain are framed as expectations as opposed to accreditation requirements. Although these focus areas were not designed to encompass all domains of HSS, we have found these useful targets for alignment and stakeholder buy-in with innovative HSS curricula and programming initiatives.

Clinical Learning Environment Review performance targets are helpful for benchmarking program performance as compared with other institutions. CLER metrics are also designed to allow for innovation, flexibility, and tailoring at the individual institution level, which enables local system adaptation. For example, although CLER establishes the expectation that residents and fellows engage in adverse event reporting, detailed specifics of how this should be achieved are not concretely delineated, and HSS programs to facilitate adverse event reporting can be designed and implemented to integrate with the needs, culture, and operations of a specific institution.

Evaluation of Individual Learners Using the Accreditation Council for Graduate Medical Education Core Competencies Framework

Whereas CLER offers a helpful framework for performance at the programmatic level, when approaching assessment of the individual learner, the ACGME Core Competencies Framework is a mainstay of evaluation of the individual GME trainee. Table 5.4 includes examples of ACGME core competencies and CLER recommendations and how these can be applied to evaluate HSS practice. All of these domains may have HSS concepts embedded within them, although systems-based practice is most directly tied to core HSS focus areas. Gonzalo et al.[34] have proposed five key priorities for advancing systems-based practice in GME, including:

- Comprehensive systems-based learning content
- Professional development continuum
- Teaching and assessment methods
- Clinical learning environments
- Professional identity as system citizens

TABLE 5.4   **Linkage of Clinical Learning Environment Review and Accreditation Council for Graduate Medical Education Milestones 2.0 to HSS Skills Assessment and Curricular Opportunity**

CLER: Safety, Quality Improvement, Teaming	Curricular Mapping Examples
Safety	Participation in institutional quality and safety training didactic offerings
	Submitting safety concerns through the institutional error reporting system
	Leading a morbidity and mortality conference using a root cause analysis framework
	Participation in a culture of safety survey
	Participation in standardized handoff processes
Health care quality	Participation in quality improvement projects
	Use of data and audit feedback to drive iterative change
	Participation in institutional quality improvement committees and clinical operations planning and implementation processes
	Engagement in projects to reduce health inequities
	Application of a health equity lens to quality improvement projects
	Use of data and audit feedback to narrow equity gaps
Teaming	Participation with team huddles to promote shared situational awareness
	Practice of interprofessional closed-loop communication in care delivery
	Recognition and engagement of the patient and family as part of the care team

TABLE 5.4   Linkage of Clinical Learning Environment Review (CLER) and Accreditation Council for Graduate Medical Education (ACGME) Milestones 2.0 to Health Systems Science Skills Assessment and Curricular Opportunity—cont'd

ACGME: Milestones 2.0	Curricular Mapping Examples and Opportunity for Assessment of the Learner
Systems-based practice 1: patient safety and quality improvement: to develop knowledge, skill, and experience with patient safety and quality improvement	Participate in identifying system errors and implementing potential systems solutions such as participating in a mortality and morbidity conference or a root cause analysis of a case During panel management in the ambulatory setting, works with electronic health record team to implement changes related to age-appropriate colonoscopy screening See safety example above See quality example above
Systems-based based practice 2: system navigation for patient-centered care	Provision of patient and family education during care transitions Facilitation of patient advancement through the system (e.g., from emergency department to ward service, ward service to intensive care unit) Create curricula related to coordination of safe transitions of care at discharge Effective patient, family, and team communication during care coordination Dissect a readmission and create processes to prevent readmissions for vulnerable population in the future
Systems-based practice 3: physician role in health care systems	Timely completion of a prior authorization request for guideline directed therapy for heart failure Discussion of choice of anticoagulation therapy with the patient includes cost, convenience, and safety Advocacy for populations and communities with health inequities Understands different medical practice models and delivery systems, and how to best use them to care for the individual patient Uses data and information technology to improve care delivery
Patient care skills 4, 5: inpatient or outpatient patient management	Review list of low-cost medications from various retail pharmacies before prescribing medications for uninsured or underinsured patient with new medications Engagement resource utilization initiatives, such as application of the Choosing Wisely campaigns Leadership of case-based discussions exploring value-based care, and cost effectiveness relevant to procedures, diagnostics, care pathways, and therapeutics
Interpersonal and communication skills 1, 2, and 3: interprofessional and team communication	Coordinate with multiple consulting teams to negotiate a shared treatment plan Participate and effectively communicate in multidisciplinary rounding with social work, case management, and nursing Document in daily progress notes with an organized explanation of the diagnosis and contingency planning if the patient acutely decompensates

CLER, Clinical Learning Environment Review; *ACGME*, Accreditation Council for Graduate Medical Education; *HSS*, Health Systems Science.

Evaluation of Health Systems Science Educators

Little is known about how to effectively evaluate HSS educators within GME. HSS educators within GME may represent attending physicians, nonphysician clinicians, health system administrators, and resident and fellow trainees. This renders knowing what, when, and how HSS concepts are taught in the clinical learning environment extremely challenging, and the logistics of disseminating and conducting educator evaluations is often not feasible because of limited resources. In our own experience surveying and conducting semistructured interviews with HSS and residency program leadership, evaluation of the educator or program by the learner is limited to nonexistent, making it difficult to know, from a trainee perspective, where gaps and deficiencies exist.

Evaluation of the Impact of Health Systems Science Programming on Patient Health Outcomes

Many of the HSS performance metrics pertaining to CLER and ACGME are structure and process metrics and focus on the individual GME program and trainee. Evaluating the impact of GME HSS initiatives on patient health outcomes is critical to understanding the effectiveness and value of integrating HSS within GME. This is also key for sustaining and spreading GME HSS initiatives and securing the resources necessary for continued programmatic infrastructure and support. Trainees can be powerful change agents and often are the team members with the most profound knowledge pertinent to how local systems can be improved.[2] More research is needed, but there is potentially significant opportunity for HSS programming in the GME environment to impact health inequities, value-based care, cost-effectiveness, and population health. This requires systems to have data accessible to trainees (through dashboards and other performance reports), such that reinforcing audit-feedback strategies can be used.

TAKE-HOME POINTS

1. The case for HSS integration in GME should be built on the Quadruple Aim, with a focus on improving population-based outcomes, mitigating health inequities, and promoting health equity.
2. Planning the HSS curriculum begins with identification of infrastructure needs and available resources through a needs assessment. The needs assessment incorporates perceived value-added viewpoints of stakeholders (e.g., learner, health system, and faculty needs) in addition to population-level health care needs, and this combines to inform the HSS framework within an institution.
3. For successful implementation of HSS curricula, a stepwise approach informed by national, standardized, shared goals and evaluation targets is needed.
4. HSS curricula in GME is supported by integration of ACGME Milestones into health system and population health needs that will challenge traditional approaches to curricula in GME.
5. GME HSS program development is crucial but must be done in conjunction with the establishment of evaluation tools to assess learners, teachers, and their impact on health outcomes. Feedback from robust assessment tools will propagate practice and culture change.

QUESTIONS FOR FURTHER THOUGHT

1. Does your institution have faculty development opportunities in HSS or education? Why is this not widely adopted?
2. What are the best ways to evaluate and assess trainees in the GME clinical learning environment when it comes to HSS skills? What are the best ways and opportunities to provide feedback?
3. What is the best way to measure the value-added of HSS program adaptation at the individual patient level and population health level?
4. How open to an HSS curricula would your institution be?

VIGNETTE 1

Your team admits a 68-year-old woman with a past medical history of cocaine use disorder, nonischemic systolic heart failure, hypertension, and diabetes mellitus type 2 who presented with shortness of breath. She has had six prior admissions in the past 7 months with similar chief concerns; usually has a course of diuresis; and is sent home with metoprolol, lisinopril, and furosemide within 5 days of admission. She now has a complicated 17-day hospital course that includes low-output cardiogenic shock. The team medically optimizes her medications during the hospitalization and starts to discuss lifestyle and diet modification. The team discusses this patient in multidisciplinary rounds, and the social worker notes she is homeless and is unclear what her insurance coverage is. She does not have family or friends and plans on "living on the streets." The medical team brainstorms on how to transition the patient safely out of the hospital.

Thought Questions

1. As the attending physician, form a list of HSS topics that could be explicitly discussed throughout the hospitalization. Form a "rounding checklist" for your team to address daily. Discuss what multidisciplinary resources and team members could have been engaged at your institution earlier in the hospitalization.
2. What is the true driver of her health care utilization? What community resources are available to help the multiple readmissions she's had?

VIGNETTE 2

As an educator, you are tasked with adding health systems science (HSS) into the curriculum but have not been given much direction. As it stands, your program holds a morning report five times a week when they go over an interesting admission from overnight. This is moderated by a faculty member or chief resident. Additionally, there are academic half days twice monthly and ambulatory didactics. In the current state, there is minimal room to add further didactic time to the residency curriculum schedule.

Thought Questions

1. What are some short-term strategies to incorporate HSS topics into the current didactic structure? In the long term (e.g., next academic year), what multilevel strategies would you have to incorporate HSS topics?
2. What would be your faculty development planning?

ANNOTATED BIBLIOGRAPHY

Gonzalo JD, Wolpaw DR, Cooney R, Mazotti L, Reilly JB, Wolpaw T. Evolving the systems-based practice competency in graduate medical education to meet patient needs in the 21st-century health care system. *Acad Med.* 2022;97(5):655-661.

Gonzalo et al. prioritize five areas of focus necessary to further evolve systems-based practices (SBP): comprehensive systems-based learning content, a professional development continuum, teaching and assessment methods, clinical learning environments in which SBP is learned and practiced, and professional identity as systems citizens.

Singh MK, Gullett HL, Thomas PA. Using Kern's 6-step approach to integrate health systems science curricula into medical education. *Acad Med.* 2021;96(9):1282-1290.

Singh et al. describe the application of Kern's six-step approach to health systems science (HSS) at the undergraduate medical education level. This paper provides clear examples, figures, and the overview of how to use a stepwise framework to apply Kern's theory to extend beyond learner-centric curricular models and apply HSS systems-minded curricular changes and curricula creation.

Thomas PA, Kern, DE, Hughes MT, Chen BY, eds. *Curriculum Development for Medical Education: A Six-Step Approach.* 3rd ed. Baltimore, MD: Johns Hopkins University Press; 2016.

The third edition of this guidebook addresses the proven six-step Kern's model for curricular development, which previously emphasized the fundamentals of writing competency-based goals and objectives and expands to incorporate milestones, entrustable professional activities, and observable practice activities. This updated version includes an awareness of new accreditation standards and regulatory guidelines with health systems science highlights in the curriculum design steps and integration approach. The expansion includes priority on interprofessional education, collaborative practice, and educational technology. The guidebook describes educational strategies that incorporate expanded pillars.

REFERENCES

1. Bodenheimer T, Sinsky C. From triple to quadruple aim: care of the patient requires care of the provider. *Ann Fam Med.* 2014;12(6):573-576.
2. Dekhtyar M, Ross LP, D'Angelo J, et al. Validity of health systems science examination: relationship between examinee performance and time of training. *Am J Med Qual.* 2020;35(1):63-69.
3. Lam PW, Wong BM. Harnessing the power of residents as change agents in quality improvement. *Acad Med.* 2021;96(1):21-23.
4. Papanicolas I, Woskie LR, Jha AK. Health care spending in the United States and other high-income countries. *JAMA.* 2018;319(10):1024-1039.
5. Milstein R, Schreyoegg J. Pay for performance in the inpatient sector: a review of 34 P4P programs in 14 OECD countries. *Health Policy.* 2016;120(10):1125-1140.

6. Blumenthal D, Abrams M. The Affordable Care Act at 10 years—payment and delivery system reforms. *N Engl J Med.* 2020;382(11):1057-1063.

7. Wilensky G. The need to simplify measuring quality in health care. *JAMA.* 2018;319(23):2369-2370.

8. Casalino LP, Gans D, Weber R, et al. US physician practices spend more than $15.4 billion annually to report quality measures. *Health Aff (Millwood).* 2016;35(3):401-406.

9. Shaheen AW, Bossenbroek Fedoriw K, Khachaturyan S. Students adding value: improving patient care measures while learning valuable population health skills. *Am J Med Qual.* 2020;35(1):70-78.

10. Centers for Medicare & Medicaid Services. *Hospital-Acquired Conditions.* Available at: https://www.cms.gov/Medicare/Medicare-Fee-for-Service-Payment/HospitalAcqCond/Hospital-Acquired_Conditions.html. Accessed April 14, 2022.

11. Centers for Medicare & Medicaid Services. *The Hospital Readmissions Reduction Program.* Available at: https://www.cms.gov/Medicare/Medicare-Fee-for-Service-Payment/AcuteInpatientPPS/Readmissions-Reduction-Program. Accessed April 14, 2022.

12. Centers for Medicare & Medicaid Services. *The Hospital Value-Based Based Purchasing (VBP) Program.* Available at: https://www.cms.gov/Medicare/Quality-Initiatives-Patient-Assessment-Instruments/Value-Based-Programs/HVBP/Hospital-Value-Based-Purchasing.html. Accessed April 14, 2022.

13. Alsubaie MA. Curriculum development: teacher involvement in curriculum development. *J Educ Prac.* 2016;7(9):106-107.

14. Lanphear JH, Cardiff RD. Faculty development. An essential consideration in curriculum change. *Arch Pathol Lab Med.* 1987;111(5):487-491.

15. Fetters ML, Duby TG. Faculty development: a stage model matched to blended learning maturation. *J Asynchronous Learn Netw.* 2011;15(1):77-86.

16. Loeser H, O'Sullivan P, Irby DM. Leadership lessons from curricular change at the University of California San Francisco School of Medicine. *Acad Med.* 2007;82(4):324-330.

17. Buring SM, Bhushan A, Brazeau G, Conway S, Hansen L, Westberg S. Keys to successful implementation of interprofessional education: learning location, faculty development, and curricular themes. *Am J Pharm Educ.* 2009;73(4):60.

18. Handler B. Teacher as curriculum leader: a consideration of the appropriateness of that role assignment to classroom-based practitioners. *Int J Teach Leadersh.* 2010;3(3):32-42.

19. Thomas PA, Kern DE, Hughes MT, Chen BY, eds. *Curriculum Development for Medical Education: A Six-Step Approach.* 3rd ed. Baltimore, MD: Johns Hopkins University Press; 2016.

20. Warman S, Pritchard J, Baillie S. Faculty development for a new curriculum: implementing a strategy for veterinary teachers within the wider university context. *J Vet Med Educ.* 2015;42:346-352.

21. Singh MK, Gullett HL, Thomas PA. Using Kern's 6-step approach to integrate health systems science curricula into medical education. *Acad Med.* 2021;96(9):1282-1290.

22. Kern DE, Thomas PA, Hughes MT. *Curriculum Development for Medical Education: A Six-Step Approach.* 2nd ed. Baltimore: The John's Hopkins University Press; 2009.

23. Moriates C, Soni K, Lai A, et al. The value in the evidence: teaching residents to "choose wisely." *JAMA Intern Med.* 2013;173(4):308-310.

24. Feldman LS. Choosing Wisely: things we do for no reason. *J Hosp Med.* 2015;10(10):696.

25. Eraut M. Informal learning in the workplace: evidence on the real value of work-based learning (WBL). *Devel Learn Organ Int J.* 2011;25(5):8-12.

26. Mitchell TD. Traditional vs. critical service learning: engaging the literature to differentiate two models. *Mich J Community Serv Learn.* 2008;14:50-65.

27. Stewart T, Wubbena Z. A systematic review of service-learning in medical education: 1998–2012. *Teach Learn Med.* 2015;27(2):115-122.

28. Strasser R, Worley P, Cristobal F, et al. Putting communities in the driver's seat. *Acad Med.* 2015;90(11):1466-1470.

29. Wilkins C, Alberti P. Shifting academic health centers from a culture of community service to community engagement and integration. *Acad Med.* 2019;94(6):763-767.

30. Petty J, Metzl JM, Keeys MR. Developing and evaluating an innovative structural competency curriculum for pre-health students. *J Med Humanit.* 2017;38:459-471.

31. Donald CA, DasGupta S, Metzl JM, Eckstrand KL. Queer frontiers in medicine: a structural competency approach. *Acad Med.* 2017;92:345-350.

32. Gonzalo J, Baxley E, Borkan J, et al. Priority areas and potential solutions for successful integration and sustainment of health systems science in undergraduate medical education. *Acad Med.* 2017;92(1):63-69.

33. Hempel E, Cooper J, Raoof E, Gonzalo J. Characterizing the prevalence and types of curricular tracks in internal medicine residency training programs. *J Gen Intern Med.* 2021;36(10):3273-3275.

34. Gonzalo JD, Wolpaw DR, Cooney R, Mazotti L, Reilly JB, Wolpaw T. Evolving the systems-based practice competency in graduate medical education to meet patient needs in the 21st-century health care system. *Acad Med.* 2022;97(5):655-661.

The Role of Interprofessional Education and Collaborative Practice in Health Systems Science Curricula

Rachel Marie E. Salas, Lisanne Hauck, Susan A. DeRiemer, and, Valerie G. Press

LEARNING OBJECTIVES

1. Define *interprofessional education (IPE)*, including its core competencies, and describe its role in health systems science (HSS).
2. Describe how interprofessional collaborative practice and teamwork are critical to achieving the Quadruple Aim.
3. Compare and contrast different strategies for developing, integrating, and tracking IPE for learners (e.g.,

do-it-yourself approach: reuse, recycle, and combine efforts and new models to teach).
4. List practical factors to consider when designing and implementing an HSS curriculum in the interprofessional space, including professional identity formation, role modeling, and techniques to bring other health professional learners together.

CHAPTER OUTLINE

Chapter Summary, 85
Introduction, 86
Implementation, 86
    Step 1: Identify the Problem, 86
    Step 2: Needs Assessment, 86
    Step 3: Learning Goals and Objectives, 87
    Steps 4 and 5: Organizational and Educational Strategies and Implementation, 88
    Step 6: Evaluation and Feedback, 89

Practical Considerations and Examples of Interprofessional Education Activities, 93
Innovations, 97
Conclusion, 99
Take-Home Points, 99
Questions for Further Thought, 100

CHAPTER SUMMARY

Teaming is one of the health systems science (HSS) foundational domains, and implementation of interprofessional education (IPE) in the health care curriculum is essential. Creating a sequential, longitudinal curriculum that builds on foundational interprofessional concepts may not be easy or intuitive. In this chapter, we present practical advice on implementing IPE into a curriculum for health care professionals. We include a basic format or template and provide structured recommendations and examples. We begin with a discussion of four significant

steps: (1) assessing the interprofessional aspects of the HSS content domain, (2) forming an interprofessional teaching team, (3) developing interprofessional training activities, and (4) selecting or developing assessment strategies and evaluation. Next, we provide definitions, terminology, and assessment tools. We then describe challenges encountered and discuss practical considerations. We also share examples from an academic institution (e.g., Johns Hopkins School of Medicine) to provide readers real activities that implement IPE. We hope that these insights and tips are useful to a variety of health care teams, faculty, administrators, and clinicians.

INTRODUCTION

Health systems science is increasingly recognized by academic institutions as the third pillar of medical education that complements basic science and clinical medicine training to ensure that health professionals apply their expertise within care systems to deliver high-value care. IPE is integral to HSS education.[1] Additionally, interprofessional care and collaboration are commonplace in major medical centers, and education in this content domain is part of the foundation of HSS.

A brief history of interprofessional collaboration will help contextualize the scenario. As early as the 1960s, health care systems recognized that medical errors often resulted from miscommunication among the health care team.[1] Many challenges existed, which were often related to the patriarchal hierarchy present in medicine at the time. Chambers et al. wrote, "Many professions had their roots entwined with status, class, and gender[2] or provide identity to their members, promoting prejudice or professional mistrust.[3] Professional isolation was perpetrated through the use of specialist language or jargon[4] or keeping individual patient records"[5] rather than sharing records or information with other specialists.

To ameliorate some of these problems, the **Association of American Medical Colleges (AAMC)** established the **Interprofessional Education Collaboration (IPEC)** group, which consisted of the AAMC and five other health care organizations involved with the formalized education of their profession, including nursing, pharmacy, public health, osteopathic medicine, and dentistry. By 2011, the IPEC created the **Core Competencies for Intercollaborative Practice** and disseminated these competencies to the health care community.[6] The four core competencies are as follow:
1. Values and ethics for interprofessional practice
2. Roles and responsibilities
3. Interprofessional communication
4. Teams and teamwork

Each competency has subcompetencies.[6] In 2016, the IPEC updated these competencies to reflect "the changes that have occurred in the health system since the release of the original report, two of the most significant of which are the increased focus on the **Triple Aim** (improving the experience of care, improving the health of populations, and reducing the per capita cost of health care) and implementation of the Patient Protection and Affordable Care Act."[6] The goals of IPE will continue to evolve and expand as they align themselves with HSS and the **Quadruple Aim** of health care, which added "improving the well-being of health care teams" as the fourth aim.[7]

Interprofessional collaboration is analogous to the concept of diverse teams working together. Other professions, most notably business and law, have discussed the benefits of diverse teams. A landmark article in the *Harvard Business Review* promoted the idea that diverse teams of workers enhance learning, creativity, flexibility, and the ability to solve problems. Diverse teams also improve job satisfaction along with personal and organizational growth. Finally, diverse teams can adapt more quickly and successfully to changing markets.[8] Medicine is an ever-changing, rapidly advancing market that requires diverse teams composed of various health professions. The health system needs diverse ideas and perspectives to enhance patient care, and those who work in the health system need to understand the value of each health profession's skill set and scope of practice.

There may be challenges to deciding when the concepts of interprofessional collaboration should be introduced in formal education. Some studies, albeit small sample sizes, suggest that a person's professional identity needs to be more securely intact before they are ready for interprofessional collaboration.[9] More thought and research are needed to dissect the idea of when and how interprofessional collaboration should be introduced. We explore the advantages and disadvantages of this point throughout this chapter.

A basic template for a longitudinally progressive curriculum could be organized into three categories: beginning learner, competent learner, and advanced learner. These could apply to undergraduate medical education (UME), graduate medical education (GME), and faculty in the medical education system. An example is provided in Box 6.1.

IMPLEMENTATION

Starting from an HSS focus, application of Kern's six steps for curriculum development, which is introduced in Chapter 1 and discussed throughout the book, is a useful framework for developing IPE activities.[10]

Step 1: Identify the Problem

The need for IPE as a key component of an HSS curriculum was discussed previously and in earlier chapters. At a given institution, additional drivers may include the need to meet accreditation standards, commitment to a comprehensive HSS curriculum, or being part of a strategy for meeting the Quadruple Aim.[7]

Step 2: Needs Assessment

Because IPE has been an accreditation requirement for both UME and GME programs, most institutions will have already identified opportunities for students and residents to participate in interprofessional training activities. However, existing interprofessional activities may not have been

---

BOX 6.1   Interprofessional Education Curricular Content by Learner Level

Beginning Learners (i.e., undergraduate medical education level)

- Didactic lectures on vocabulary, concepts, roles, and responsibilities of each health care profession (e.g., the scope of practice).
- Practical experience with different professions; students spend time in various roles.
- Interaction with other student health care professionals and discussions of specific clinical cases designed to highlight the collaborative nature of medical care.

Competent Learners (i.e., graduate medical education level)

- Residents or in-training professionals collaborate on "social rounds," which discuss the total care of each patient. Medical, nursing, pharmaceutical, psychosocial,

case management, nutrition, and other specialties are involved in discussions of each patient.

- Transition of care discussions (e.g., discharge planning) during which teams collaborate to ensure that all aspects of a patient's care are established and a follow-up plan is created.

Advanced Learners (i.e., faculty and practicing clinician level)

- Attend and lead social rounds and transition care discussions attended by the competent learner groups (i.e., graduate medical education learners).
- Attend two continuing medical education events per year on topics related to interprofessional education, health systems science, communication skills, team buildings, and other topics.

---

developed from an HSS perspective, and it may be necessary to determine how best to integrate them into the overall HSS curriculum. Conversely, activities focused on HSS domains may need to be modified to incorporate an interprofessional perspective.

Each of the core functional, foundational, and linking domains of HSS and each level of the health system (micro, meso, macro) involves contributions from different mixes of professions. For instance, in addressing medication errors at the micro level, the key professions might include medicine, pharmacy, and nursing. For students to understand the impact of social constructs on health, they may need to have the perspectives of public health, social work, and law. Institutional assessments of structures and processes that affect health outcomes can be tapped to identify potential interprofessional perspectives to integrate into the training of physicians. Process mapping, flow charts, and critical driver analyses can all be used to identify professions to include in a team focused on a particular aspect of HSS or a team that will work on a comprehensive interprofessional HSS curriculum.

Step 3: Learning Goals and Objectives

After the professions have been identified, the task becomes identifying specific individuals and recruiting them into HSS teaching teams. This is the group that will be actively engaged in setting the goals and objectives as well as the organizational and educational strategies. In most cases, these people will also play a role in implementation and responding to evaluation data. The added complexity of developing activities that involve different professions and often different institutions means that attending to creating a guiding coalition and developing a shared vision

and strategy (Kotter steps 2 and 3) should be explicitly addressed in developing interprofessional curricula.

Institutional factors may smooth the initial step of identifying potential team members. Medical schools located within universities that train multiple professions may create teams within their institution. If there is an office of IPE, the groundwork to identify individuals who have both the skills and the interest in interprofessional health systems teaching may have already been completed. For educators in medical schools without associated training programs for other professionals, practical strategies include drawing on professional networks, including those of other professionals providing clinical care at training sites, and contacting nearby institutions to identify key educators. In considering potential collaborators, it is essential to determine interests and skills in IPE and practice as well as expertise in their field. Low-stakes initial roles such as giving a guest lecture, participating on an interprofessional panel, or serving as a consultant or guest expert during an existing IPE activity are ways to engage potential partners who can progress to more substantial contributions, including engagement of their students.

A particular aspect of forming educational teams to address the Institute for Healthcare Improvement's goals of improving patient experience and population health is how to involve patients and community members. Patient and family input at all stages of the training can best be obtained by the inclusion of representatives on the interprofessional team. Reaching out to community advocacy groups and patient advisory boards for help identifying appropriate individuals can ensure that training activities not only include patient perspectives but also address health system issues of importance to them. Patient perspectives can also be incorporated into specific activities through in-person or recorded interviews, feedback on student recommendations, and inclusion of their stories in case studies.

Significant structural challenges may impede participation by even faculty members who are interested in IPE. These need to be identified and addressed. These include any institutional requirements for memoranda of understanding or limitations on who can teach or supervise students. Support from deans and department chairs is essential for obtaining dedicated release time or inclusion of interprofessional team membership in assigned responsibilities. Also important are recognitions relevant to professional advancement, both internal and external. Approaches may include the development of an interprofessional educator certification or award, facilitating faculty presentations at national meetings, and structuring activities to facilitate publication. Budgets for interprofessional training activities may require accessing external funding.

An effective interprofessional faculty team, after it is formed, needs time to develop trust; resolve potential conflicts (professional and personal); address issues of diversity, equity, and belonging; develop a shared mental model; and establish team norms. For instance, how does the team address conflicts in the scope of practice or reimbursement? Does team leadership reflect traditional health system hierarchies? Is the team membership reflective of the student and patient populations, and if not, how will they ensure the inclusion of diverse viewpoints? What is required for effective communication? Monitoring the process of forming a high-functioning IPE team and modeling the problem-solving processes required can inform students' development of practical training activities. It is important to schedule opportunities for faculty to interact in both formal and informal sessions as part of team formation, and over time, these interactions can facilitate connections that support not only the original activity but also expanded interprofessional initiatives and faculty development. Regular faculty team meetings also enhance sustainability in the face of faculty turnover by providing support and mentoring for new faculty.

The need to coordinate across professional training programs is the only difference between interprofessional curricular activity planning and the development of any other curriculum. Addressing the basic questions of who, what, when, and where may require additional compromise, creativity, and flexibility when dealing with multiple professions. For instance, in determining which students should participate, it is necessary to account for the different durations of training programs. A second-year advanced practice nurse or a dietetic intern is at a different point in their professional development than a second-year medical student, and each may have had different levels of preparation related to HSS content. Pairing students at different levels may require targeted preparation to bring everyone to a common starting point. Monitoring student evaluation of the appropriateness of the activity and their ability to participate fully may suggest a need to restructure the teams.

Setting shared educational objectives for interprofessional training is most manageable when dealing with critical thinking and teaming skills, which are similar across professions. It can be harder to define shared knowledge objectives. For instance, a medical student, a physical therapy student, and a social work student all need an understanding of what happens when a patient breaks a hip, but the specific knowledge each needs is quite different. Teams may decide that there will be interprofessional shared objectives as well as ones that are profession specific. Most of the HSS domains are covered in the training programs of other health professions, but the depth of coverage and the specific content differ across programs.[7] Medicine has led the way in defining HSS content and characterizing it as an essential pillar of medical training. Integrating HSS objectives into interprofessional training activities may require explaining this structure to both faculty and students from other professions and determining how the HSS objectives for a given activity are formulated within the other profession's curricula.

Steps 4 and 5: Organizational and Educational Strategies and Implementation

The added complexity of educational activities that engage students and faculty from multiple professional training programs means that the details of implementation need to be incorporated as educational strategies are selected. The time and effort investment is significantly greater than for an activity that needs to meet the needs of only one set of learners, and the risks of failure are greater. The level of institutional recognition and support for these activities may be crucial in determining success and sustainability. When beginning a new partnership for IPE, it is also important to start with activities that have a high probability of success to generate short-term wins (Kotter step 6) that reward partner investment and can be used to justify the required institutional investments.

A variety of formats can be used for delivering interprofessional content, and the MedEdPORTAL's Interprofessional Collection and the Interprofessional Educational Collaborative are good sources for tested materials. Commonly used formats for 1- to 4-hour sessions include case studies, team-based learning, and simulations. Formats for multiple sessions can include a shared educational module, for instance, on structural and social determinants of health or assigning an interprofessional team of students to a common clinic location and time. Finally, quality improvement projects at the community or clinic level may involve an entire elective or multiple semesters. Because there is no aspect of medicine that does not involve professional collaboration, interprofessional training has the potential to be incorporated into most areas of medical education. There are, however, practical constraints that may limit the strategies available to a particular program. Three of these constraints are discussed next.

Will the Activity Be Required, Optional, or Extracurricular?

Interprofessional activities can be required for all students in the formal curriculum, an option within the curriculum that only some students may select, or an extracurricular element of the informal curriculum, an option that the Liaison Committee on Medical Education (LCME) also monitors. A universally required activity may need to be structured differently to accommodate larger groups of students and may preclude some formats. Whether an activity is required, optional, or extracurricular also impacts student engagement in complex ways. Students participating in a graded, required activity may focus on meeting a grading rubric and may be more likely to question the applicability of the activity to their training than students who have chosen to participate. How an activity is framed becomes even more important when incorporating it into clerkships and residency training. A required clerkship activity may need to be repeated four or more times each year, and it may need to be designed such that it can be used at different clinical sites, which may not be accessible to the existing interprofessional partners and which may have unique logistical constraints. For example, residency programs must balance work-hour limitations and the demands of clinical care delivery.

When Will the Activity Occur?

In addition to determining time in the curriculum, IPE demands finding times that work for students with packed classes and clinical schedules that may vary within a day or across the academic year. Some activities can be done in the evenings or on weekends to reduce conflicts, but this will not work for all students. If possible, teams should identify dates and times before academic calendars are finalized and aim for consistency from one year to the next.

Will Participants Meet in Person or Virtually?

There are a number of factors to consider when deciding whether interprofessional training activities will be in person or virtual. Virtual activities tend to cost significantly less because there is not a need to pay for facilities, audiovisual equipment, food, and transportation. Virtual meetings also facilitate participation by students in online educational programs who may be located across the country and allow for institutions that are geographically distant to collaborate. Virtual training has several drawbacks, including Internet connectivity issues and most significant, more difficult personal interactions because of limited ability to send and receive nonverbal communication signals.[1] Some activities may be amenable to hybrid formats that allow students to meet in person before or after online work sessions. Virtual interprofessional meeting spaces provide a third option that are increasingly familiar to today's students.

Step 6: Evaluation and Feedback

Interprofessional education within the context of HSS should be evaluated to ensure learners and clinical team members are achieving educational and clinical team goals and objectives. A common approach to evaluation is to assess knowledge, attitudes, and skills. For general information on curriculum evaluation, see Chapters 3 and 7 for information on selecting an evaluation paradigm and specifically with respect to applying Kirkpatrick's New World Model of evaluation.[10-12]

With respect to specific frameworks and tools for the evaluation of IPE within and external to HSS, numerous ones are available (Table 6.1). A handful of systematic reviews has evaluated these tools, often within a specific specialty, and for the most part, no single comprehensive tool has been identified for complete IPE assessment.[13,14] In one systematic review of prelicensure IPE, 39 tools were identified, and knowledge was the most commonly assessed outcome.[13] Another systematic review evaluated IPE outcomes for pharmacy education and found 36 relevant tools, with no one comprehensive tool identified.[10] Because no one tool will be the ideal IPE assessment tool for all settings and even within specific IPE curricula, this section of the chapter summarizes the types of assessments, the outcomes assessed, and the learners and clinicians who are the focus of the assessments and tools (see Table 6.1). These assessment tools were identified from a review of the literature, including the systematic reviews[13,14] cited earlier and from the National Center for Interprofessional Practice and Education.[15]

Learner (Pre- and Postlicensure)

Assessment tools for learners participating in IPE range from those that focus on attitudes or self-efficacy, those that focus on knowledge or skills, and those that aim to be more comprehensive. Furthermore, whereas some of these tools are agnostic to the IPE learners, other tools focus on single or multiple learners from specific clinical training programs. Some of these tools simultaneously evaluate

TABLE 6.1 Interprofessional Education Assessment Tools

Domain	Tool	User/Use	Setting	Example Use
Learner Focused				
HSS specific with IPE domain(s)	NBME HSS Examination	Learners, medical students	Multiple	For use among medical students to assess HSS domains including IPE
Multiple tools and domains	Almoghirah H, et al.[12]: 39 prelicensure IPE assessment tools summarized in a systematic review	Learners, general	Multiple	For use evaluating prelicensure students in IPE
	Shrader et al.[13]: 36 IPE assessment tools for pharmacy students summarized in a systematic review	Learners, pharmacy	Multiple	For use evaluating pharmacy students in IPE
Attitudes and behaviors of student learners	Interprofessional Attitudes Scale (IPAS)	Learners, general	Curricula, clinical rotations	Course directors obtain students' self-assessed attitudes of IPE before and after an IPE intervention
	Students Perceptions of Interprofessional Clinical Education Revised (SPICE-R)	Learners, general	Curricula, clinical rotations	Course directors obtain students' self-assessed perceptions of IPE before and after an IPE intervention
	Attitudes Toward Health Care Teams Scale (ATHCT)	Learners, professional practice, general	Curricula, clinical rotations	Course directors obtain students' self-assessed attitudes of IPE before and after an IPE intervention
	Student Perceptions of Physician-Pharmacist Interprofessional Clinical Education (SPICE-2)	Learners, physician–pharmacist student dyads	Curricula, clinical rotations	Third-year medical students paired with pharmacy students on IPE curricula and clinical rotations
Knowledge of student learners	IPEC Competency Self-Assessment Tool	Learners, professional practice, general	General	Preclinical students complete these self-assessments to aid course directors in curricula planning

TABLE 6.1	Interprofessional Education Assessment Tools—cont'd			
Domain	**Tool**	**User/Use**	**Setting**	**Example Use**
Skills of student learners	TeamSTEPPS Team Assessment Questionnaire and Team Performance Observation Tool (TAQ-TPOT)	Learners, general	Clinical, simulation	Preclinical learners participate in simulation training for rapid response teams; the instructors use the TAQ-TPOT to evaluate learners' communication, leadership, and team processes
	Team Observed Structured Clinical Encounter (TOSCE)	Learners, general	Clinical	Learners participating in team-based clinical care can be assessed as individuals and as a team
	Interprofessional Collaborative Competencies Attainment Survey (ICCAS)	Learners, professional practice, general	Pre- and postinterventions	An IPE intervention is rolled out, and the ICCAS is used to assess interprofessional student learners pre- and postintervention implementation
	Teamwork Assessment Scale (TAS)	Physicians in training	Simulation	Second-year medical students are being trained for their participation in clinical wards, and the instructors use TAS to evaluate their teamwork skills in a simulated setting
Learning environment	Assessment for Collaborative Environments (ACE-15)	Professional practice	General	Faculty and course directors need to rapidly assess clinical teams for placement of preclinical learners in clinical IPE settings
Professional Practice				
Attitudes and behaviors of clinicians in practice	Team Climate Inventory (TCI)	Professional practice	General	Health care management team wants to measure the team's climate
	Healthcare Team Vitality Instrument (HTVI)	Professional practice	General	An IPE team is interested in learning about individual team members' perceptions of team-based communication, engagement, support, among other factors

Continued

TABLE 6.1   Interprofessional Education Assessment Tools—cont'd

Domain	Tool	User/Use	Setting	Example Use
Skills of clinicians in practice	Assessment of Interprofessional Team Collaboration Scale (AITCS)	Professional practice	General	A team wants to measure actual collaboration, not just perceptions of individuals' ability to collaborate
	Team Decision Making Questionnaire (TDMQ)	Professional practice	General	A health care team comprised of interprofessional team members aims to evaluate their ability to make team-based decisions
Both Student and Professional Practice				
Attitudes and behaviors of students and clinicians in practice	Interprofessional Socialization and Valuing Scale (ISVS-21)	Students, professional practice	General	Pre- and postevaluation of students and practicing clinicians in clinical practice
	Individual Teamwork Observation and Feedback Tool (iTOFT)	Students, professional practice	General	A comprehensive review of an IPE intervention for preclinical and clinical students as well as junior faculty
Patient Perspective				
Impact on patients	Patients Insights and Views Observing Teams Questionnaire (PIVOT)	Patients, general	Clinical	Patients on a clinical ward are invited to evaluate all team members including students and those in professional practice
	Communication Assessment Tool-Team (CAT-T)	Patients, physicians	Clinical	Patients being seen in an ambulatory clinic

HSS, Health systems science; *IPE,* interprofessional education; *NBME,* National Board of Medical Examiners.

learners and clinicians in practice, and others are solely focused on evaluating the learners.

The National Board of Medical Examiners has a Health Systems Science Examination that assesses, in part, IPE.[16] Some assessment tools evaluate across multiple domains. As mentioned previously, a couple of systematic reviews were completed that identified numerous tools with variable attention to knowledge, skills, and attitudes.[13,14]

Attitude-specific assessment tools regarding interprofessional practice include the Interprofessional Attitudes Scale (IPAS), the Students Perceptions of Interprofessional Clinical Education Revised (SPICE-R), and the Attitudes Toward Health Care Teams Scale (ATHCT).[17-19] IPAS is a 27-item tool that can be used across health care learners to assess students' self-reported beliefs and attitudes about interprofessional care collaboration.[17] A shorter three-item tool that also assesses students' perceptions of interprofessional team practice is SPICE-R.[18] ATHCT focuses on learners and practitioners' beliefs about the care quality provided by the care teams and the attitudes of these individuals regarding the physicians' central authority role, also known as "physician centrality," in these care teams.[19] There are also discipline-specific assessment tools such as the Student Perceptions of Physician-Pharmacist Interprofessional Clinical Education (SPICE-2) tool.[20]

Assessments of learner knowledge in preparation for student placement, curricula development, and so on also exist.[21,22] These include the IPEC Competency Self-Assessment Tool, a tool that assesses students' self-reported competency and self-efficacy and can help with curricula planning.[21]

There are numerous tools to assess learner skills, including[23-26] TeamSTEPPS Team Assessment Questionnaire and Team Performance Observation Tool (TAQ-TPOT),[23] Team Observed Structured Clinical Encounter (TOSCE),[24] Teamwork Assessment Scale (TAS),[25] and the Interprofessional Collaborative Competencies Attainment Survey (ICCAS).[26] The TAQ-TPOT is a 43-item questionnaire that can be used for the real-time clinician or simulation-based settings to observe learners' participation in teams, including domains of communication and leadership, among others.[23] The TOSCE includes two seven-item tools designed for assessment of learners' individual and team performance in clinical settings.[24] The TAS is a 14-item tool designed to train and evaluate preclinical medical students in simulation-based settings on teamwork.[25] The ICCAS is a 20-item tool that can be used before and after IPE interventions to assess team-based competencies.[26]

The Assessment for Collaborative Environments (ACE-15) is a 15-item tool that aims to aid with a rapid assessment of the quality of interprofessional care teams to aid with student or learner placement.[22]

Professional Practice

For health care teams wanting to evaluate their vision and support for innovation, among other measures, educators should consider using the Team Climate Inventory (TCI), a 38-item self-report tool.[27] If teams want to evaluate their "vitality," they can use the Healthcare Team Vitality Instrument (HTVI). This 10-item tool can be used across a wide range of clinicians and clinical training settings.[28,29] For health care teams interested in evaluating IPE skills, tools such as the 37-item Assessment of Interprofessional Team Collaboration Scale (AITCS)[29] or the 19-item Team Decision Making Questionnaire (TDMQ) can be used.[30]

Both Learner and Clinician

One tool, the Interprofessional Socialization and Valuing Scale (ISVS-21), can be used to evaluate students and practicing clinicians' interprofessional socialization. The tool uses self-report to measure individuals' attitudes, behaviors, and beliefs before and after an IPE intervention.[31] Another tool, the Individual Teamwork Observation and Feedback Tool (iTOFT), can be used among multiple different IPE learners, from pre-clerkship to clerkship students to early-career faculty and clinicians. This tool measures 10 behaviors across four domains, including teamwork, leadership, patient safety, and shared decision-making.[32]

Patient Assessment of Interprofessional Education

There are also tools that evaluate the impact of IPE on patients. Two of these tools include the Patients Insights and Views Observing Teams Questionnaire (PIVOT)[33] and the Communication Assessment Tool-Team (CAT-T).[34] The PIVOT is a 16-item tool that allows patients to evaluate team members' communication, coordination, and interactions, among other behaviors.[35] The CAT-T is a patient satisfaction survey focused on team-based communication.[36] Of note, both the PIVOT and the CAT-T were initially tested for use in the emergency department setting.

PRACTICAL CONSIDERATIONS AND EXAMPLES OF INTERPROFESSIONAL EDUCATION ACTIVITIES

It can be challenging to integrate HSS content into curricula, which includes embedding IPE and collaborative practice into the culture. Institutions may find it cumbersome to incorporate formal or structured IPE into their curricula across the educational continuum, especially in the context of limited time. So how might an educator teach and address IPE across such a wide array of professions? Should they start at a basic, fundamental level, introducing vocabulary, concepts, skills, and core competencies in the beginning years of the health professions curricula? At what stage of training is it appropriate or best for learners to have the clinical application of these skills and knowledge? How can a curriculum build on its foundation, enhance **spiral learning**, and encourage continual growth and exploration of HSS topics? These are some of the challenges to IPE implementation and buy-in. Most IPE begins as students enter school in year 1 of their health professions program. Students learn in a didactic manner about topics such as health care components, scope of practice, roles and responsibilities, skills and tasks, and the professional requirements necessary to obtain a degree in their chosen field. In the early years of schooling, knowledge is typically acquired in a concrete, methodical way. At the same time, learners are beginning to explore the journey of professional identity formation, which evolves and expands as they develop their sense of self.

One often encountered challenge is that although IPE may be explicitly placed into the UME/GME curriculum, there is no guarantee that this is what is being modeled in the clinical environment. If learners do not observe interprofessional collaboration in clinical practice, then there is disconnect, even disappointment. Learners participate in clinical experiences and encounter mentors and role models who they strive to emulate in and outside their profession. It is well described that as learners progress, knowledge is often obtained in the hidden curriculum in the clinical setting, typically by observing clinicians. Often these clinicians are physicians who were not formally trained in IPE and may model traditional hierarchy where the physician is the team leader. Although some of these role models may embody and role model an interprofessional approach, not all may to the same degree, or learners may not be there to witness it because interprofessional collaboration may happen at times when the learner is not present. Bedside rounding is variable by the service or unit, health care team, and the physician with whom the learner may be directly working. Additionally, there may not always be a structured interprofessional approach during clinical rotations or experience.

For example, a student may attend an outpatient sleep neurology clinic in an interprofessional sleep center where physicians, medical assistants, nurses, respiratory therapists, sleep technologists, and sleep behavioral psychologists all work together. However, the student may be assigned to work with a specific physician preceptor, and although this physician may also practice with an interprofessional team, the physician may not explicitly role model this in front of the student and instead may focus more on the physical examination, presenting, and note writing with the student. One recommendation to consider for this preceptor in this example would be to have the student see two patients and do a presentation and examination. The preceptor should then ensure that the student also be present when the preceptor speaks with the respiratory therapist on the team about one of the patients. Many times, the physician will have a meaningful discussion and obtain the perspective from the respiratory therapist to provide better care. However, in the patient room, the preceptor may say in front of the student, "I will have you (the patient) speak with the respiratory therapist to address the issues with your continuous positive airway pressure device," which may appear to be not explicitly collaborative but instead prescriptive.

Teaching and precepting physicians often have limited time in their clinical practices at baseline. Added responsibilities to teach during clinics can be overwhelming. However, having educational leaders such as clerkship directors help preceptors prioritize what they are going to teach, role model interprofessional behaviors, and identify who from the health care team the learner will engage with in clinical practice can be beneficial. Speaking with course and clerkship directors to help preceptors better frame their activities as interprofessional can not only be beneficial by explicitly showcasing this to students but also helpful to the school of medicine by having an accurate map of where and how IPE is formally being taught. Clerkship and course directors have recognized that IPE

varies and often create interprofessional activities to allow learners to experience interprofessional practice in a more explicit manner. See Table 6.2 for some examples at one institution.

Bringing together learners from various health professions requires intentional organization and forethought. Health professions schools and programs within the same enterprise often have unique academic schedules and course requirements, and schools may not be physically located near each other, making it challenging to identify times when learners can come together to engage in interprofessional learning. Alignment of learners in their training so that they are at the same level from the perspective of clinical knowledge, so to speak, to engage in the educational activity is another challenge. Furthermore, many academic programs include IPE activities as a graduation requirement and may house an IPE activity either in isolation as a stand-alone educational activity or may include the activity as part of a course. Although on the surface, such flexibility is allowing each health professions program to categorize an IPE curricular activity as to how they see fit in their overall academic program, the complexities of such can result in inconsistencies across learners involved.

For example, in Baltimore, Maryland, the Interprofessional Collaborative composed of Johns Hopkins University School of Medicine, Johns Hopkins University School of Nursing, Johns Hopkins Bloomberg School of Public Health, and Notre Dame of Maryland University School of Pharmacy have a large IPE event series with four IPE events (two in the first year and two events in the second year of the programs) anchored on the four overall IPEC competencies. The first event is a social event to promote interprofessional connection and introductory IPE concepts. In this real example, the schools of medicine (SOM), nursing (SON), pharmacy (SOP), and public health (SPH) join together to host the four events. Although each school designates one or more of these events as a graduation requirement, there is some variability. The SOM and SPH opt to have the social event optional for their students, but the SOP and SON require it. Furthermore, the SPH only requires one IPE event centered around public health for their students. The SON and SOP require all four events to receive credit, but the SOM requires three of the events.

Adding to the complexity is that each school may have different grading specifications. For example, the SOM requires attendance and engagement during the activity and completion of pre- and postevent surveys to receive credit, which equates to a grade of "pass" for the event as a standalone academic requirement. In contrast, the SON includes the event(s) as part of a formal credit IPE course that results in a grade for the course with a tiered grading system. Furthermore, the SOP may require the first two events as

TABLE 6.2 Examples of Interprofessional Education Preclinical and Clinical Curricular Activities at Johns Hopkins School of Medicine

	Course	Activity	Participants
Pre-clerkship phase	IPE events	Two sessions in year 1 and two sessions in year 2 (total of four sessions); the first session is a social and introductory event	Learners: medical students, nursing students, public health students, pharmacy students Faculty: nurse, pharmacist, physician, public health expert, social worker
	Topics in Interdisciplinary Medicine (TIME): Patient Safety course	Multiple experiences over three half days, including small group sessions, simulations, and lectures	Learners: medical students Faculty: nurse, pharmacist, physician, infection control practitioner, human factors engineer, teamwork expert, safety coach
	TIME High-Value Healthcare course	Students work in small groups led by pharmacists	Learners: medical students Faculty: pharmacist, physician
	Pain and Opioids course	Session on the potential role for nonphysicians in the management of acute and chronic pain, recognizing how physicians can collaborate with other team members to manage pain	Learners: medical students Faculty: physician, nurse, pharmacist, physical therapist, psychologist, policymaker
	Interprofessional elective	Health Systems Science: Interprofessional Collaboration to Improve Medication Safety	Learners: nursing, medical students Faculty: nurse, pharmacist, physician medical resident or fellow
	Interprofessional elective	Health Systems Science: Fostering Future Leaders for Interprofessional Practice	Learner: medical students Faculty: nurse, pharmacist, physician
	Interprofessional elective	Ethical and policy challenges in the era of COVID-19: implications for clinical practice, research, and public health	Learners: medical students Faculty: ethicist, physician

Continued

TABLE 6.2   Examples of Interprofessional Education Preclinical and clinical Curricular Activities at Johns Hopkins School of Medicine—cont'd

	Course	Activity	Participants
Clerkship phase	Transition to the wards	Interprofessional shadowing with hospital staff activity	Learners: medical students Faculty: nurse, social worker, chaplain, respiratory therapist, patient advocate, physical and occupational therapists, hospital administration leaders
	Neurology and Psychiatry clerkship	Caregiving and Dementia: An Interprofessional Didactic with a Patient Caregiver	Learners: medical students Faculty: caregiver, nurse, physician, patient advocate
	Women's Health clerkship	Scenarios on breastfeeding experience, lactation, intimate partner violence scenario, postpartum depression scenario	Learners: medical students Faculty: lactation specialist, social worker, psychologist, physician
	Internal Medicine clerkship	Discharge skills for medical students session	Learners: medical students Faculty: pharmacist, nurse, case manager
	Advanced Ambulatory clerkship	Students accompany a Johns Hopkins Home Care registered nurse in person to perform patient continuity of care across transitions (hospital to home) Advocacy experience: students spend 1 day with an organization learning how individuals and organizations are working to address health and health care inequities at the local, state, or national level	Learners: medical students Faculty: home care nurse, care management coordinator, health care advocate
	Interprofessional Clinical elective	The Hospital: Walk in Their Shoes	Learners: medical students Faculty: nurse, social worker, chaplain, respiratory therapist, patient advocate, physical and occupational therapist, hospital administration leader

TABLE 6.2 Examples of Interprofessional Education Preclinical and clinical Curricular Activities at Johns Hopkins School of Medicine—cont'd

	Course	Activity	Participants
Extracurricular	Interprofessional Interest Group	Teaming Up for High-Value Care: Interprofessional Student Interest Group goal is to create an interprofessional interest group for health professions students	Learners: nursing students, medical students Faculty: physician, nurse, pharmacist
	Interprofessional Death Café	Interprofessional Death Café: the principles include an agenda-free discussion about death and dying with the aim of normalizing end-of-life discussions in an accessible, open, and confidential environment The goal is to create space for students and faculty to share fears and experiences about encountering death (professionally and personally) and to listen to the unique perspectives of their colleagues	Learners: medical students, public health students, nursing students Faculty: nurse, physician, public health expert
	AfterWards program	AfterWards is an interprofessional narrative medicine program at Johns Hopkins designed to illuminate stories of healing for the healers	Learners: medical students, public health students, nursing students, clinician in any health profession; open to anyone

IPE, Interprofessional education.

part of a course like the SON but may also require other events in year 2 as a stand-alone graduation requirement in which students would receive a pass for participation and completing postevent surveys. In contrast, the SPH requires the event for graduation but does not offer a grade of any sort and only documents participation. Such variability in how an IPE activity may be incorporated into each of the health professions schools and how students earn credit for the activities may result in the perception of unbalance. If one school places more value by means of providing a grade or by requiring more of the events, this may send the message that the other schools do not value IPE to the same degree.

On the other hand, a stand-alone medical school that does not have another health professions school in proximity may have different challenges. In the time before virtual educational opportunities were the mainstay, such schools would have found themselves in a problematic situation, often requiring innovative strategies to bring learners from different health professions together in person. However, now that the virtual education renaissance has emerged, academic programs are finding themselves in the throes of many new, previously unavailable options.[35] Currently, educational programs can invite learners from other health professions programs in other institutions out of their city, state, and country.

INNOVATIONS

The COVID-19 pandemic has provided the opportunity for innovation. Virtual IPE platforms can be developed to provide a collaborative space for students not only across local institutions but also nationally and even globally. For Johns Hopkins University's IPE social event for networking and connection discussed in the previous section, the four schools came together to create their own virtual campus hosted on Gather Town, an online platform. The 2-hour session consisted of a human bingo and IPE scavenger hunt in the customized IPE town in Figs. 6.1 and 6.2 with five large halls, an auditorium, and a large green space. Educational leaders from each of the four schools (SON, SOM, SOP, and SPH) attended the event to welcome, mingle, and interact with students. The virtual IPE world will serve as a place to hold subsequent IPE activities and is the meeting place for the IPE directors. Currently, some of the IPE electives that share students among the schools use the IPE virtual space as their campus. Educators at Johns Hopkins also created an IPE interest group that plans to use this virtual space as well.

At the postlicensure level, at Johns Hopkins, we (chapter author R. Salas along with interprofessional peers at Johns Hopkins) have created an IPE GME Distinction Program composed of two tracks, the Health Systems Science and the Health Humanities Track. A parallel HSS Distinction Track is also being piloted at Lewis Katz School of Medicine at Temple University in the Internal Medicine Residency program.[36] Johns Hopkins and Temple HSS educators are collaborating to implement and study the track in two similar but personalized ways at two institutions. Although still in pilot form, this program plans to expand to include other postlicensure learners (e.g., pharmacy residents and doctor of nursing practice students) in the upcoming year. One example of IPE development from the faculty perspective is the recognition and establishment of an IPE faculty exemplar program so that faculty from across schools can be invited or selected to be role models for IPE events and activities. Such an initiative can lead to the building of an IPE and HSS faculty-centered community that provides development, recognition, and nurturing for faculty. This was achieved by one of the coauthors of this chapter (R. Salas) who co-created an interprofessional faculty professional development strengths coaching program (Becoming A Health Professions Super Model Program) that was open to all health professionals with the institutions and beyond in which faculty can obtain personalized coaching relating to their strengths and professional identity formation. Strengths coaching provides a unique way to celebrate individuals beyond their health profession, skill set, and past experiences to promote personal and team development. This strengths-based approach has now been implemented into several other

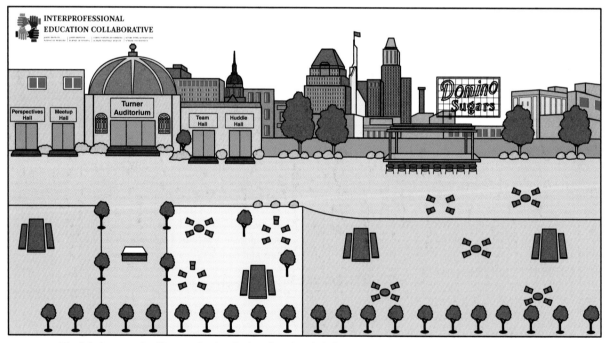

Fig. 6.1 A customized interprofessional education virtual platform. Johns Hopkins School of Medicine, Johns Hopkins School of Nursing, Johns Hopkins Bloomberg School of Public Health, and Notre Dame of Maryland University School of Pharmacy worked with Association Management Solutions to develop and customize a virtual campus on Gather Town to bring the four schools together. Each school has one hall that is theirs, and the Turner auditorium has a Zoom link for hosting large sessions. The Gather Town platform allows private spaces for individuals to meet one on one, in small groups, or in larger groups. There are games imbedded as well as a poster for each profession in each room. (From Association Management Solutions.)

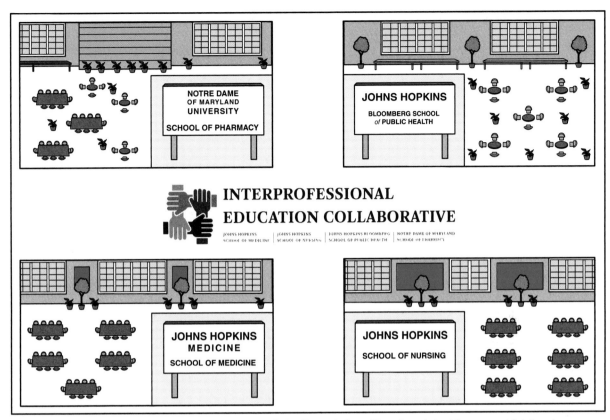

Fig. 6.2 Interprofessional education halls on the Gather Town platform. (From Association Management Solutions.)

IPE programs across the IPE collaborative at Johns Hopkins (e.g., Health Systems Science: Fostering Future Leaders for Interprofessional Practice elective course; School of Education Master of Education for Health Professions program; Health Systems Science GME Distinction Track).

CONCLUSION

For many medical schools, IPE had been occurring in a variety of ways in the curriculum long before HSS was established as the third pillar of medical education. With the formalization of HSS, IPE has been rebranded and now falls under "teaming" as one of the foundational domains in the HSS framework. Governing medical organizations such as the LCME, Accreditation Council for Graduate Medical Education, and Accreditation Council for Continuing Medical Education have all embraced the importance of IPE and collaborative practice ensuring that teaming is a core foundational domain for current and future physicians.

TAKE-HOME POINTS

1. Teaming falls under the HSS umbrella as a foundational domain, making the implementation of IPE in the health care curriculum essential.
2. Governing bodies encourage and include IPE and collaborative practice as important for health professionals.
3. Various models and activities have been implemented in health professions schools and now, with advancement in virtual education, new IPE opportunities are possible.
4. Many assessments to measure teaming (and IPE) are available and should be considered when developing and implementing IPE in the curriculum.

QUESTIONS FOR FURTHER THOUGHT

1. How can medical educators continue to promote IPE and teaming into the culture so that it is ingrained in all aspects of medical education and clinical practice?
2. What are new opportunities to develop faculty to role model interprofessional collaborative practice in their day-to-day duties?
3. Now that virtual platforms are widespread, what are the opportunities for you to further develop IPE at your institution?

VIGNETTE 1

A medical school faculty member has been charged with developing longitudinal interprofessional training activities in health systems science (HSS) for undergraduate medical education. The faculty member assembles a working group with members from multiple institutions and health professional training programs. The team members share their program goals and details of their curricula over the course of several meetings and agree to begin with planning an initial activity that will address medication errors, transitions of care errors, and the Interprofessional Education Collaborative's core competencies. Before implementation, one training program drops out because of changes in the key faculty member's responsibilities.

Additionally, some programs opt to make the activity optional as opposed to required which impacted the makeup of the interprofessional teams. The team leader is concerned about maintaining the momentum of the working group, considering the challenges encountered in this first effort.

Thought Questions

1. How should programs balance required, optional, and extracurricular opportunities for interprofessional education (IPE) and practice within the HSS curriculum?
2. What institutional structures and processes are needed to develop and sustain IPE collaborations in HSS?

VIGNETTE 2

A university has multiple clinical training programs, including medicine, nursing, pharmacy, and social work. An interprofessional curriculum committee is formed to develop interprofessional education curricula for their clinical students. The aims of the curricula involve an intervention that would allow the learners to simultaneously provide value-added roles on clinical rotations. The committee recognizes they will need to evaluate the effectiveness of this curricular intervention across all learners.

Thought Questions

1. What evaluation or assessment tools would be useful to measure the learners' attitudes, behaviors, and skills?
2. Can the same tools be used across all learners, or will there need to be learner-specific tools?

ANNOTATED BIBLIOGRAPHY

Interprofessional Education Collaborative. *Core Competencies for Interprofessional Collaborative Practice: 2016 Update.* <https://hsc.unm.edu/ipe/resources/ipec-2016-core-competencies.pdf.>; 2016. Accessed 15.04.22.
Being familiar with the four Interprofessional Education Collaborative core competencies for interprofessional collaboration is essential for any health systems science (HSS) educator developing, implementing, or participating in interprofessional education (IPE) in a health professions curriculum.
Joint Accreditation. <https://www.jointaccreditation.org>; Accessed 15.04.22; *National Board of Medical Exa miners Subject Examinations Program Guide.* <https://www.nbme.org/sites/default/files/2021-04/NBME_Subject_Exam_Program_Guide_2021.pdf>; Accessed 15.04.22.

The Joint Accreditation establishes the standards for education providers to deliver continuing education planned by the health care team for the health care team.
National Board of Medical Examiners Subject Examinations Program Guide. <https://www.nbme.org/sites/default/files/2021-04/NBME_Subject_Exam_Program_Guide_2021.pdf>; Accessed 15.04.22.
The National Board of Medical Examiners has published a Health Systems Science Examination that evaluates across a range of health systems science domains, including IPE. Assessment of IPE interventions can help institutions understand the added value of IPE educational opportunities for preclinical and clinical students across health disciplines, including team-based learning, self-efficacy, communication, and other important skills.

REFERENCES

1. Joint Accreditation. <https://www.jointaccreditation.org>; Accessed 15.04.22.
2. Barr H. Interprofessional education: the fourth focus. *J Interprof Care.* 2007;21(2):40-50.
3. Carpenter J. Interprofessional education for nursing and medical students. Evaluation of a program. *Med Educ.* 1995;29:265-273. <https://doi.org/10.1111/medu.1995.29.issue-s1>.
4. Pietroni PC. Towards reflective practice—the languages of health and social care. *J Interprof Care.*1992;6(1):7-16.
5. Chambers A, Clouder L, Jones M, Wickham J. Collaborative health and social care, and the role of interprofessional education. In: Porter SB, ed. *Tidy's Physiotherapy.* 15th ed. Churchill Livingstone; 2013:23-39. doi:10.1016/B978-0-7020-4344-4.00002-X."
6. Interprofessional Education Collaborative. *Core competencies for Interprofessional Collaborative: 2016 Update.* <https://ipec.memberclicks.net/assets/2016-Update.pdf>; 2016. Accessed 15.04.22.
7. Bodenheimer T, Sinsky C. From triple to quadruple aim: care of the patient requires care of the provider. *Ann Fam Med.* 2014;12(6)573-576.
8. Thomas DA, Ely RJ. Making differences matter: a new paradigm for diversity. *Har Bus Rev.* 1996;74(5):79.
9. Stull CL, Blue CM. Examining the influence of professional identity formation on the attitudes of students towards interprofessional collaboration. *J Interprof Care.* 2016;30(1):90-96.
10. Singh MK, Gullett HL, Thomas PA. Using Kern's 6-step approach to integrate health systems science curricula into medical education. *Acad Med.* 2021;96(9):1282-1290.
11. Institute of Medicine. *Health Professions Education: A Bridge to Quality.* Washington, DC: The National Academies Press; 2003.
12. Kirkpatrick JD, Kirkpatrick WK. *Kirkpatrick's Four Levels of Training Evaluation.* Alexandra, VA: Versa Press; 2016.
13. Almoghirah H, Nazar H, Illing J. Assessment tools in pre-licensure interprofessional education: a systematic review, quality appraisal and narrative synthesis. *Med Educ.* 2021;55(7):795-807.
14. Shrader S, Farland MZ, Danielson J, Sicat B, Umland EM. A systematic review of assessment tools measuring interprofessional education outcomes relevant to pharmacy education. *Am J Pharm Educ.* 2017;81(6):119.
15. *National Center for Interprofessional Practice and Education.* Assessment and Evaluation. <https://nexusipe.org/advancing/assessment-evaluation>; 2021. Accessed 15.04.22.
16. *NBME National Board of Medical Examiners (NBME) Health Systems Science Examination.* <https://www.nbme.org/sites/default/files/2021-04/NBME_Subject_Exam_Program_Guide_2021.pdf>; Accessed 15.04.22.
17. Norris J, Carpenter JG, Eaton J, et al. The development and validation of the interprofessional attitudes scale: assessing the interprofessional attitudes of students in the health professions. *Acad Med.* 2015;90(10):1394-1400.
18. Dominguez DG, Fike DS, MacLaughlin EJ, Zorek JA. A comparison of the validity of two instruments assessing health professional student perceptions of interprofessional education and practice. *J Interprof Care.* 2015;29(2):144-149.
19. Heinemann GD, Schmitt MH, Farrell MP, Brallier SA. Development of an attitudes toward health care teams scale. *Eval Health Prof.* 1999;22(1):123-142.
20. Fike DS, Zorek JA, MacLaughlin AA, Samiuddin M, Young RB, MacLaughlin EJ. Development and validation of the student perceptions of physician-pharmacist interprofessional clinical education (SPICE) instrument. *Am J Pharm Educ.* 2013;77(9):190.
21. Dow AW, DiazGranados D, Mazmanian PE, Retchin SM. An exploratory study of an assessment tool derived from the competencies of the interprofessional education collaborative. *J Interprof Care.* 2014;28(4):299-304.
22. Tilden VP, Eckstrom E, Dieckmann NF. Development of the assessment for collaborative environments (ACE-15): a tool to measure perceptions of interprofessional "teamness." *J Interprof Care.* 2016;30(3):288-294.
23. Baker DP, Amodeo AM, Krokos KJ, Slonim A, Herrera H. Assessing teamwork attitudes in healthcare: development of the TeamSTEPPS teamwork attitudes questionnaire. *Qual Saf Health Care.* 2010;19(6):e49.
24. Lie D, May W, Richter-Lagha R, Forest C, Banzali Y, Lohenry K. Adapting the McMaster-Ottawa scale and developing behavioral anchors for assessing performance in an interprofessional team observed structured clinical encounter. *Med Educ Online.* 2015;20:26691.
25. Kiesewetter J, Fischer MR. The teamwork assessment scale: a novel instrument to assess quality of undergraduate medical students' teamwork using the example of simulation-based ward-rounds. *GMS Z Med Ausbild.* 2015;32(2):Doc 19.
26. Archibald D, Trumpower D, MacDonald CJ. Validation of the interprofessional collaborative competency attainment survey (ICCAS). *J Interprof Care.* 2014;28(6):553-558.
27. Anderson NR, West MA. Measuring climate for work group innovation: development and validation of the team climate inventory. *J Organiz Behav.* 1998;19:235-258.
28. Upenieks VV, Lee EA, Flanagan ME, Doebbeling BN. Healthcare Team Vitality Instrument (HTVI): developing a tool assessing healthcare team functioning. *J Adv Nurs.* 2010;66(1):168-176.
29. Orchard CA, King GA, Khalili H, Bezzina MB. Assessment of Interprofessional Team Collaboration Scale (AITCS): development and testing of the instrument. *J Contin Educ Health Prof.* 2012;32(1):58-67.
30. Batorowicz B, Shepherd TA. Measuring the quality of transdisciplinary teams. *J Interprof Care.* 2008;22(6):612-620.
31. King G, Orchard C, Khalili H, Avery L. Refinement of the Interprofessional Socialization and Valuing Scale (ISVS-21) and development of 9-item equivalent versions. *J Contin Educ Health Prof.* 2016;36(3):171-177.
32. Thistlethwaite J, Dallest K, Moran M, et al. Introducing the individual Teamwork Observation and Feedback Tool (iTOFT): development and description of a new interprofessional teamwork measure. *J Interprof Care.* 2016;30(4):526-528.

33. Henry BW, Rooney DM, Eller S, Vozenilek JA, McCarthy DM. Testing of the Patients' Insights and Views of Teamwork (PIVOT) survey: a validity study. *Patient Educ Couns.* 2014; 96(3):346-351.

34. Makoul G, Krupat E, Chang CH. Measuring patient views of physician communication skills: development and testing of the Communication Assessment Tool. *Patient Educ Couns.* 2007;67(3):333-342.

35. Berman NB, Durning SJ, Fischer MR, Huwendiek S, Triola MM. The role for virtual patients in the future of medical education. *Acad Med.* 2016;91(9):1217-1222.

36. Shah Pandya D, Salas RME. *Health Systems Science Graduate Medical Education Distinction Tract: A Tale of Two Academic Medical Institutions.* <https://cdn.flowcode.com/prodassets/Poster_Health_Systems_Science_Graduate_Medical_Education_Distinction_Track.pdf?ts=1644513210560663687>; 2021 [poster presentation]; <https://flowcode.com/p/unPxTtxBw?fc=0>.

Sustainability in a Health Systems Science Program: Assessment, Evaluation, and Continuous Improvement

Daniel A. Novak, Beth A. Hawks,* F. Lee Revere, and Ronan Hallowell

LEARNING OBJECTIVES

1. Identify elements of sustainability planning as applied to educational programs.
2. Describe how models of change can be used to sustain and improve health systems science (HSS) education.
3. Generate a longitudinal evaluation plan for an HSS educational program.
4. Summarize the structures and processes needed for a robust continuous quality improvement program to sustain successful HSS curricula and programs.

CHAPTER OUTLINE

Chapter Summary, 104
Introduction: Sustainability through Planning, Assessment, and Evaluation, 104
Sustainability as a Dynamic Process, 104
Planning for Sustainability with Kotter's Model of Change, 104
   Evaluating the Sustainability of Health Systems Science Programs, 105
Evaluating, Improving, and Sustaining Health Systems Science Programs with Logic Models, 106
Program Evaluation for Effectiveness, Sustainability, and Cultural Change, 107
   Applying Kirkpatrick's Levels of Evaluation to Health Systems Science Curricula, 107
Quality Improvement and Long-Term Sustainability, 110
   Outcomes, 110

Processes, 110
Structures, 110
Structural Challenges to Continuous Quality Improvement, 111
   Curricular Features: Time, Sequence, Changes, and Explicit Integration with Other Portions of the School Curriculum, 111
   Gaining and Building Buy-in from Faculty, Preceptors, Leadership, and Students: A Commitment to Institutional Mission and Culture and Commitment of Executive Leadership to the Curriculum, 111
   Clinical Learning Environment, 111
   Faculty Time, Faculty Development, and Technology, 112
   Institutional Hierarchy and Reporting Relationships, 113
   External Resources, 113

---

*The contents, views, or opinions expressed in this publication or presentation are those of the authors and do not necessarily reflect official policy or position of Uniformed Services University of the Health Sciences, the Department of Defense, or Departments of the Army, Navy, or Air Force. Mention of trade names, commercial products, or organizations does not imply endorsement by the U.S. Government.

CHAPTER OUTLINE—cont'd

Process Challenges to Continuous Quality
  Improvement, 113
Outcome Challenges to Continuous Quality
  Improvement, 113
Using Continuous Quality Improvement Processes to
  Develop Sustainability, 114

Conclusion, 115
Take-Home Points, 116
Questions for Further Thought, 116

CHAPTER SUMMARY

This chapter reviews several key features of long-term sustainability for health systems science (HSS) education interventions, proceeding from definitions and theories of sustainability to the use of assessment, evaluation, and **continuous quality improvement (CQI)** processes to help guide planning and responses. The chapter concludes with additional long-term considerations for sustainability. Although these factors are typically considered at the end of a project's design, this chapter will help medical educators see that sustainable HSS educational programs (curricula, learning strategies, learner assessment, and program evaluation) require deep planning from the beginning. To achieve long-term change, medical educators must begin with the end in mind.

INTRODUCTION: SUSTAINABILITY THROUGH PLANNING, ASSESSMENT, AND EVALUATION

Sustainability is the process of ensuring that the gains achieved via an initiative are maintained beyond the life of a given project.[1] Ensuring the sustainability of successful HSS education initiatives may require realignment of the entire instructional system to support the new changes. The kinds of systemic changes necessary to support HSS education beyond the life of a single project can be complicated, may be costly, and are often unanticipated.

SUSTAINABILITY AS A DYNAMIC PROCESS

The processes that support **sustainability** have been studied for more than three decades with models of sustainability that operate at very different units of analysis. This long conceptual history can make finding the right model of sustainability planning difficult for individuals responsible for change management in HSS education. In a 2018 review of sustainability in evidence-based interventions in public health, Shelton et al.[2] found that many initiatives conceptualize sustainability as an outcome that can be

reached or an objective that can be completed. The authors noted sustainability should instead be understood as a dynamic process of adapting and responding to new demands over time. By applying this conceptual framework of sustainability as a dynamic process to HSS curricula, schools and programs can create adaptive educational initiatives that are responsive to changes in educational systems, health systems, and the health care environment. It also helps educators better respond to challenges and barriers as they arise. For example, programs do not have to succumb to the commonly reported phenomena of "voltage drop" (or decrease in benefits as sustainability increases) or program drift (in which benefits decrease as programs drift from strict implementation protocols) when they remain in an adaptive stance.

This section presents two approaches used in medical education and in other health care change management contexts. The first approach is a change management model developed by Kotter[3] that frames sustainability as a dynamic process of change management. Kotter's framework provides a clear understanding of the trajectory of change processes that lead to sustainable change over time and is described in more detail in Chapter 1. The second approach is the Program Sustainability Assessment Tool (PSAT), a framework to help assess program sustainability over time.[4] The PSAT looks at a range of features that are crucial for programmatic success, and the instrument can easily be used on a routine basis to assess sustainability at different points in time. Used together, Kotter's framework and the PSAT can help HSS program developers, instructors, and administrators ensure they have all the necessary tools for planning and assessing their change initiatives in flexible ways that respond to the dynamic demands of HSS curriculum implementation. The following sections describe each approach in more detail.

PLANNING FOR SUSTAINABILITY WITH KOTTER'S MODEL OF CHANGE

Understanding change as a long-term, dynamic implementation project can help HSS faculty and administrators plan for the multiple changes they will encounter in implementing and sustaining HSS curricula. The choice of implementation framework can have a profound impact on the success of the project depending on environmental, personnel, and institutional factors that must be understood from the outset.[5] Kotter's model of change has frequently been used in studies of health care organizational improvement.[6] However, programs that implement Kotter's model often neglect the sustainment phase, including two key, final steps: (7) consolidate gains and (8) anchor new approaches in the organizational culture. As Kotter notes, reducing effort before achieving sustainable changes can lead to losses in performance, returns to baseline, or outright chaos. The creation of an unsustainable HSS educational program may cause administrators, faculty, and students to question the value of the program. Given these high stakes, it is essential to recognize the importance of sustainability planning to the success of HSS programs and align the necessary people and resources to support these programs for the long term.

The Kotter model may be especially useful in mapping the growth of a sustainable HSS program because each phase involves multiple stakeholders. The initiation phase requires buy-in and input from educational and health system leaders and grows to encompass more of the institutional community over time. The implementation phase grows to include still more of the community as curriculum developers, instructional designers, and faculty become involved in the development process. Finally, in the sustainment phase of the model, the program grows to become part of the institutional culture itself. When this goal has been achieved, HSS programs are not just perceived as an additional box to check but will become an essential part of how students, residents, and physicians are trained.

Evaluating the Sustainability of Health Systems Science Programs

After building on Kotter's conceptual foundations, it is important to periodically check to ensure the HSS program has the necessary resources to accomplish its goals. This process requires input from leaders, faculty, and learners. For this reason, it is useful to align the sustainability process with a validated tool that has been developed to work specifically within health care. The PSAT from George Washington University[4] provides a strong theoretical framework for understanding and evaluating sustainability in change management interventions. The PSAT divides the necessary sustainability "ingredients" into eight components that are applicable to a range of HSS education initiatives (Box 7.1).

The PSAT has been subjected to validation in a number of public health domains and programs. Luke et al.[7] conducted a validation study representing 252 public health programs in chronic disease domains such as tobacco control, diabetes, obesity, and oral health. This study found that despite domain differences within health care, the tool was able to successfully demonstrate relationships with important program and organizational characteristics.

BOX 7.1 The Program Sustainability Assessment Tool's Eight Components of Sustainability

Environmental support: The program has supportive internal and external climates, with champions who can obtain resources, support from administrators, and support from the public.

Funding stability: The funding base for the program is consistent, diversified, and reinforced by policy.

Partnerships: The program cultivates connections with stakeholders in the community who are invested in its success.

Organizational capacity: The program has sufficient internal support, backing, and resources that support its activities; is well integrated into the organization's operations; and has adequate staff and material resources.

Program evaluation: The program is the subject of periodic evaluation that informs planning; documents outcomes; and provides short-, intermediate-, and long-term evidence that the program works.

Program adaptation: Managers take action to help the program adapt in ways that ensure its ongoing effectiveness through periodic reviews of the evidence base, adaptation of new strategies, responsiveness to changes in the environment, and pruning of ineffective components

Communication: The program engages in strategic communication with stakeholders and the public to maintain support, communicate the program's values, generate awareness and interest, and demonstrate value.

Strategic planning: The program uses processes that guide its direction, goals, and strategies to plan for future needs; clearly outline roles and responsibilities; and maintain adaptive readiness.

(Data from Schell SF, Luke DA, Schooley MW, et al. Public health program capacity for sustainability: a new framework. *Implement Sci.* 2013;8(1).)

Similarly, the use of the framework in a variety of health care settings has allowed other organizations to develop best practices around the use of the tool itself.[8] The PSAT can be used in a variety of ways to support HSS education initiatives, including as a 360-degree program evaluation tool to conduct periodic snapshots of sustainability for institutional reports and as a means of spotting problems in programs before they become catastrophic. By combining Kotter's model for sustainable change and the PSAT, HSS educators will ensure their change efforts are planned and evaluated with sustainability in mind.

EVALUATING, IMPROVING, AND SUSTAINING HSS PROGRAMS WITH LOGIC MODELS

Successful HSS program implementation and sustainability requires clear articulation of the intended program goals, outcomes, and benefits during the initiation and implementation phases of Kotter's model. **Logic models** are tools used to plan, improve, and analyze the sustainability of change at more granular levels (e.g., department, program, or initiative). A brief description of logic models and an HSS curricular logic model example are included in Chapter 3.

When curriculum developers use logic models to guide their change processes they can align planned changes and their outcomes more precisely. This planning approach provides a structured methodology for ensuring curriculum development, deployment, and evaluation lead to the expected outcomes. Logic models provide micro-level details regarding the necessary resources, process steps, actions, and expected outcomes in advance of program implementation. "Logic models depict the theory of change that drives the program and describe the resources available to implement the program, as well as the rationale behind the effort."[9]

In their simplest form, a logic model links inputs to outputs and outputs to outcomes. Inputs are the resources necessary to start a program such as an HSS curriculum program, including things such as curricula, faculty, time, and classroom space. Outputs are the activities or delivery of the educational experience (e.g., the active learning activities delivered by the instructors). Finally, outcomes are the expected results from the content delivery in terms of the changes in performance, behavior, or organizational culture that developers plan to see from their students.

Irwin et al.[9] describe three types of logic models that may support the development of an HSS program depending on the needs of the logic model developers. The first type, a theory-approach logic model, provides an overview of the program (i.e., HSS curriculum) and can be used for external stakeholders. The second model, an activities logic model, focuses on the actions needed to deploy the program and the logical sequence of actionable items. In this model, the action steps are directly linked to the expected outcomes. The third type is the outcomes-approach logic model. This model is similar to the activities in the second type but with a stronger focus on outcomes and the relationship of process steps to achieve the outcomes. The selected approach in developing an HSS curriculum logic model should be specific to the institution and the intended use of the model. Regardless of the type of logic model chosen, the development steps are similar.

After selecting a type of logic model, developers can follow the four-step process to devise a logic model for their program.

- **Step 1:** Assess available resources (inputs), including materials, support, and the knowledge needed to support the activities required to develop an HSS curriculum. This includes a gap analysis of existing, related HSS content and activities.
- **Step 2:** Delineate the activities (actions) necessary to create or deliver the HSS curriculum. Activities include content development, faculty buy-in, learner input, and curriculum committee approval.
- **Step 3:** Identify the expected tangible and measurable outputs of activities. Note that outputs do not demonstrate if the intending outcomes were achieved as they are process-oriented results. Examples are the number of lectures provided, the types of content included, or the number of students trained. The outputs are achievable through the activities listed in the logic model.
- **Step 4:** Determine the expected short- and long-term outcomes of outputs. For example, a short-term outcome of an HSS curriculum may be learner-driven, such as demonstrated knowledge in quality improvement (QI). A long-term outcome may require learners to use their QI knowledge to improve a clinical outcome during residency or fellowship. Alternatively, a long-term outcome might include feedback from residency sites noting that program graduates consider cost when making clinical decisions. The short- and long-term outcomes are unique to each HSS curriculum because they reflect an educational program's unique resources, activities, and outputs.

For more resources on developing a logic model, access the Institute of Educational Sciences' *The Logic Model Workshop Toolkit*.[10] The toolkit is designed to help practitioners learn the purpose and utility of logic models and includes detailed instructions on the appropriate steps and use of logic models for program evaluation.

Evaluating the success of an HSS program and identifying opportunities for improvement is key to program sustainability. If a team uses a logic model for planning and implementing an HSS curriculum, the logic model becomes a helpful tool to retrospectively assess the effectiveness of their efforts. Gaps in actual and expected outcomes can be mapped to the outputs, activities, and resources. Failure to achieve long-term outcomes is caused by unmet short-term outcomes. Similarly, if there is a shortfall in meeting the short-term outcomes, critical evaluation should be given to the HSS curriculum outputs. Either the outputs are unmet, or they are not aligned to the outcomes. In the latter case, careful evaluation of the outputs may reveal poor alignment between outputs and outcomes, suggesting a need for improvement in output selection or attainment. The links between the outcomes, outputs, activities, and resources should be evaluated to determine the root cause for unmet outcomes. The HSS program logic model can be a tool for identifying necessary changes in the curriculum going forward if teams use a CQI approach.

The sustainability of a successful HSS program requires ongoing measurement, evaluation, and modification. As resources change, the logic model can identify gaps between materials, support, and knowledge needed, and what is available. Similarly, sustainability requires an ongoing review of the HSS curricular activities and mapping within the logic model. Content modification, faculty changes, and accreditation standards are some of the many reasons why the activities listed in the HSS curriculum logic model may shift. Subtle changes in these activities may ultimately impact the short- or long-term outcomes. Programs and schools are encouraged to establish an HSS committee, supported by the curriculum committee, which provides a formal structure for regular assessment of the components of the HSS curricular logic model. It is through these routine assessments that the HSS curriculum will be continuously improved and indefinitely sustained.

Ridinger et al.[11] developed a logic model to summarize themes from their qualitative study of Vanderbilt University Medical Center residents and faculty from multiple specialties describing HSS-successful entering residents, including inputs, learning activities, outputs, and outcomes (Fig. 7.1). This model could be used to inform an HSS program logic model for undergraduate medical education (UME) or graduate medical education (GME).

PROGRAM EVALUATION FOR EFFECTIVENESS, SUSTAINABILITY, AND CULTURAL CHANGE

In ensuring sustainability, evaluation is the collection of processes applied to curricula and programs to ensure they are providing value to all stakeholders. According to Kirkpatrick and Kirkpatrick[12] there are three major reasons to evaluate educational programs: (1) to find opportunities to improve the program, (2) to maximize the transfer of learning to other aspects of an organization, and (3) to demonstrate the value of the program learning outcomes to the organization. **Program evaluation** is also a critical component in the improvement of program services.[13] Conducting this kind of evaluation can include asking probing questions about whether the program is meeting the needs of all stakeholders, whether there are any wasted or inefficient efforts in the program, and if there are unintended consequences of a program.

Although these questions are central to an effort's success, the evaluation of educational programs is sometimes treated as an afterthought instead of as a key part of the design and implementation process. This can lead to a range of negative consequences, such as unclear mission achievement. Developing a longitudinal evaluation plan helps to assure stakeholders that the program is working well in all domains of interest.

Health systems science is a unique medical science discipline in that it encompasses sets of concrete skills (e.g., navigating electronic health records and conducting CQI projects) as well as more complex, long-term dispositional developments (e.g., becoming an effective "systems citizen," i.e., having a professional identity linked to a commitment to HSS knowledge and equipped with structural competencies). Although some skills can be learned and assessed immediately through tools such as objective structured clinical examinations (OSCEs), learners may require years of enculturation and exposure to develop more complex attitudes, values, and dispositions. This is especially true for UME programs in which students are also engaged in professional identity formation.

Applying Kirkpatrick's Levels of Evaluation to Health Systems Science Curricula

Examining the quality of HSS programs requires a longitudinal approach because each measure of program quality provides only a snapshot of the total picture. Evaluators must ensure that they are conducting their program evaluations at the correct level to ensure their program outcomes are being met rather than completing evaluations at convenient times. The Kirkpatrick New World Model of evaluation framework,[12] also described in Chapter 3, can help evaluators go beyond surface level characteristics of program performance. The four Kirkpatrick model levels or outcome domains (reaction, learning, behavior, and results) can help program developers to purposefully sample program performance data in ways that support continuous improvement and sustainability from learning environments to performance environments. Although these levels are frequently shown in numerical order, they should be used

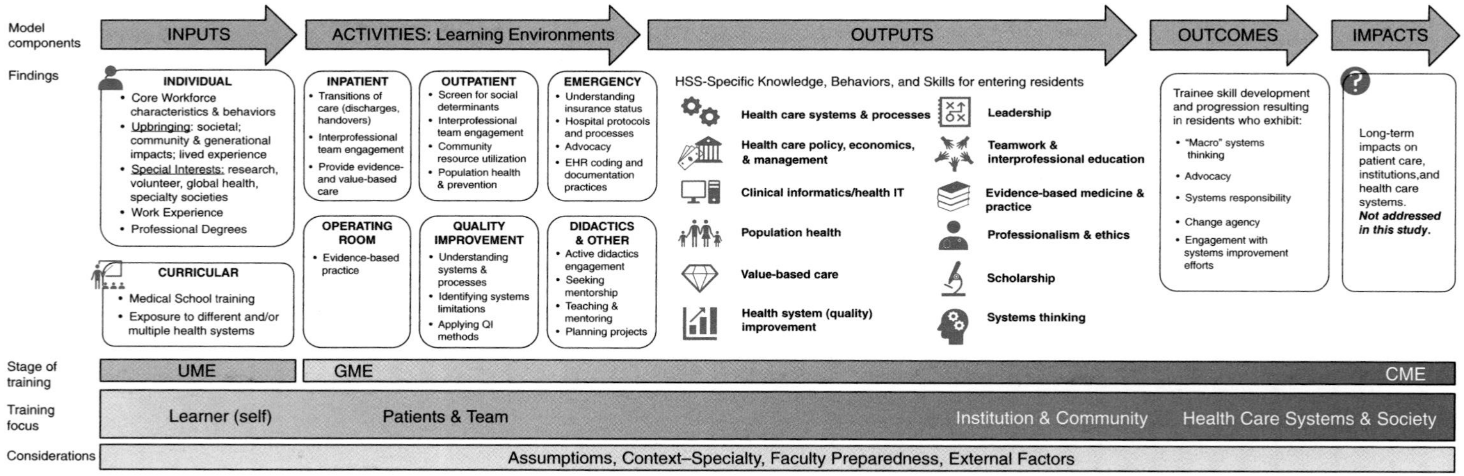

Fig. 7.1 Logic model for health systems science–prepared entering residents. *CME*, Continuing medical education; *EHR*, electronic health record; *GME*, graduate medical education; *HSS*, health systems science; *QI*, quality improvement; *UME*, undergraduate medical education. (Reproduced with permission from Ridinger HA, Bonnet K, Schlundt DG, Tekian A, Riddle J, Lomis KD. Defining successful practice within health systems science among entering residents: a single-institution qualitative study of graduate medical education faculty observations. *Acad Med*. 2021;96(11 suppl):S126-S135.)

in reverse order to promote alignment between a program's results, behavior, learning, and reactions. By proceeding in reverse order, HSS program evaluators ensure that they are truly beginning with the end in mind.

Kirkpatrick Level 1: Reactions

Historically, program evaluators have relied heavily on the use of student satisfaction surveys to determine the effectiveness of their programs. Although asking students about their experience has some value in the evaluation process, these measures are subject to variation due to racial and gender biases,[14] student motivation,[15] time of day, and other nonprogrammatic conditions. Other studies have indicated that learners are poor judges of the effectiveness of learning experiences relative to their perception of its value.[16]

Additionally, medical students often have strong feelings about the perceived relevance of content to their needs, but these feelings may be influenced by institutional demands such as exams, OSCEs, and their beliefs about what doctors should know.[17] In a 2020 study of medical students' end-of-course evaluations, Gonzalo et al. found that although students perceived the relevance of HSS to their professional identity formation, tensions existed between their perceived value of HSS content relative to the value of basic and clinical science curricula. Further, students preferred content with testable facts as opposed to content that required complex understanding and deep engagement with ideas. If program evaluators limit their HSS program analysis to the students' perspective, they may erroneously believe their programs are not meeting the needs of stakeholders.

Kirkpatrick Level 2: Learning

A deeper evaluation of HSS program effectiveness must proceed beyond learner satisfaction to measurable outcomes of learning. Chapter 2 proposes a set of HSS competencies which educators can use when defining learning outcomes. Because HSS content is complex, it may not be possible to test more global learning outcomes in standardized conditions such as examinations and OSCEs (particularly in domains such as systems thinking or policy evaluation). As Gonzalo et al.[18] note, assessment of HSS attitudes, knowledge, and skills may leverage existing assessment strategies but may also require the development of new observational tools or assessment conditions that ideally assess learners' knowledge in the field. They note that learner "assessment methods related to teamwork, quality, safety, and evidence-based practice include multiple-choice exams, knowledge application tests, work product ratings, simulation-based tools, indirect observation methods (e.g., peer assessment, multisource feedback), and direct observation of clinical activities." The authors also warn that use of unvalidated or homegrown HSS assessments should be eschewed in favor of collaborative research into validated assessment tools. However, assessment of student learning in these ways cannot be the conclusion of a program evaluation process because student learning in HSS domains is not the end of the line. Student learning must lead to changes in behavior and organizational culture.

Kirkpatrick Level 3: Behavior

Although reactions and learning are important to a program's outcomes, HSS programs must also fundamentally lead to changes in behavior. Tables 2.1 and 2.2 summarize the intersections of HSS to existing national frameworks, curricula, and accreditation requirements from groups such as the American Medical Association (AMA), Association of American Medical Colleges (AAMC), and the Accreditation Council for Graduate Medical Education (ACGME). Although the development of these standardized expectations is ongoing and the HSS competencies in Chapter 2 will require modification over time, Ridinger et al.[11] found it was possible to arrive at consensus about how an HSS-prepared learner might function upon entering a GME learning and practice environment. In residency, students who were well-prepared to become systems citizens were identified by a range of specific behaviors that were agreeable to attendings as well as fellow residents. By creating a similar kind of consensus, other HSS programs may find it easier to develop evaluation tools that allow evaluators to track how effectively their program prepares learners to exhibit changes in behavior in their organizational context.

Kirkpatrick Level 4: Results

Whereas accreditors, universities, and other medical education stakeholders highly value student learning as measured on assessments, program evaluators in HSS are concerned with program impacts beyond individual learner changes. That is, after learners have successfully completed their HSS coursework assessments, program evaluators should investigate how these students' presence in the health system change the way that the system operates. For example, Gonzalo, et al.[19] found that the integration of HSS content could lead to the development of new kinds of professional identities (e.g., systems citizen) that can lead to broader systemic transformation. Furthermore, Davis and Gonzalo[20] identify several ways that the implementation of HSS curricula may lead to improved integration between medical schools and the communities they serve. Measuring the impact of HSS programs on the quality of care provided to communities should be an essential component of any evaluation plan but would be invisible to stakeholders if program evaluation concludes at Level 1, Level 2, or Level 3.

In selecting the right paradigms for an evaluation program and following the changes from a program beyond the classroom, evaluation can play a central role in bringing HSS into a sustainable relationship with the rest of the curriculum. However, to bring about real change in health systems, the evaluation process must remain part of the dynamic, ongoing evolution of a sustainable HSS program.

QUALITY IMPROVEMENT AND LONG-TERM SUSTAINABILITY

Building on the logic model and using a CQI approach, HSS leaders can apply Donabedian's framework for measuring the quality of health care (structure, process, and outcomes) to measuring the quality (i.e., success) of education interventions.[21,22] This framework, briefly mentioned in Chapter 3, can be used at both the macro- (program, curriculum) and the micro-level (e.g., activity, assignment, lesson, course). Donabedian[21] argued that "a good structure increases the likelihood of a good process, and a good process increases the likelihood of a good outcome." Unlike the logic model, which is intended for curriculum development and stakeholder engagement, Donabedian's framework provides a simple, user-friendly approach for implementing a robust process for CQI and thus sustainability. Because the focus is on achieving and sustaining the HSS curriculum, this section uses a backward design approach and starts with outcomes.

Outcomes

Donabedian[21] describes **outcomes** as the effects on patients and populations, which includes knowledge and behaviors. In this context, the desired outcomes are the effects (knowledge and behaviors) and effectiveness that the HSS curricula will have on learners and the impact on their patients, health care delivery, or the health care system. To identify the short-term outputs and long-term outcomes that the institution has for the HSS curriculum, medical educators should refer back to the program's logic model where the outputs and outcomes are delineated. To measure these outcomes, educators should also establish incremental annual goals to promote attainable successes based on the resources of the institution to meet the outcomes. HSS curriculum teams should outline the goals in a SMART (specific, measurable, achievable, relevant, and time-based) format to help to clarify these incremental goals.

It is tempting to develop an exhaustive list of goals for a program in an effort to achieve an ideal state. However, this comes with increased risk that resources (human and financial) at institutions will be diluted and few or none of the goals will be achieved. We recommend medical educators prioritize programmatic goals, ensure they work with each other (or at least not against one another), and focus on a concise list of goals. For example, if a logic model states that graduates will demonstrate cost-effective decision-making, perhaps a reasonable goal is that 50% of graduates will report that they consider the cost of a diagnostic test, treatment, or medication when making decisions or recommending a course of action. Another feasible goal may be that all graduates will report discussing costs when counseling patients on expensive treatments or medications.

Processes

In clinical care, **processes** are the activities or steps in performing routine work in caring for patients. In this context, they are the activities needed for faculty to develop and deliver the curricula and to ensure its long-term sustainability. Similar to the inputs and activities in a logic model, processes should be clearly defined by their purpose, frequency, and ownership. However, in the logic model the inputs and activities were defined such that specific outputs would be achieved. Using Donabedian's framework we recommend processes are evaluated as a part of CQI. Relevant questions might include the following:

- When will annual goals be set?
- When will the curriculum be reviewed?
- Who will review the curriculum and provide feedback?
- How will feedback need to be incorporated?
- How will student feedback be collected, analyzed, and used to improve the curriculum?

Structures

Much like a logic model outlines the necessary inputs for an HSS curriculum, **structures** in Donabedian's framework are the resources (e.g., people, equipment, supplies) required to complete the clinical activities or process steps to achieve the desired clinical outcomes. Similarly, medical educators must consider resource availability. These resources include formal and informal communication, leadership structures, and faculty and staff. Donabedian supported the notion that organizational structure drives the ability to perform the desired processes. Using the Donabedian framework for CQI allows HSS curriculum developers to take a systems approach to improvement because it requires consideration of the internal and external environment. A program's ability to improve and sustain an HSS curriculum is dependent on an institution's unique structure. This unique structure undoubtedly shapes quality assurance and improvement activities.

Donabedian's framework of structure, process, and outcomes is well-researched in health care. It provides a systems-view for CQI and reminds us that each HSS curriculum or program will be unique to the system in which it resides. As such, the mechanisms for monitoring, improving, and sustaining the program will also be unique.

Implementing a comprehensive HSS program in UME and GME is advantageous to the health care system and those it serves. HSS programs disseminate and advance knowledge necessary for health professionals to achieve the Quadruple Aim: improving the quality of care, patient outcomes, and health care provider well-being as well as minimizing overall costs.[23] Collectively working toward these goals can significantly affect patients and the health care system (e.g., private payers, public payers, and care delivery institutions). With these gains come notable challenges for the CQI and sustainability of HSS programs. Evaluation and subsequent CQI ensure the program is meeting its mission and strategic goals or outcomes. Sustainability reflects the ability to maintain the program over time, which can be achieved by routinizing the HSS program into UME and GME institutions. Program sustainability can be influenced by active championing, stakeholder support, showing clear benefit to institutions and patients, and the program's alignment with the organizational mission.[24,25] Below we use the Donabedian framework of structure, process, and outcome described earlier to categorize some of the common CQI challenges and suggestions to promote sustainability.

STRUCTURAL CHALLENGES TO CONTINUOUS QUALITY IMPROVEMENT

Structure refers to the environment and resources needed to complete the *process* step, which is needed to get the desired *outcomes* when it comes to building and maintaining an educational program.[26] When applying this lens to CQI and sustainability of an HSS program, program owners need to pay close attention to institutional buy-in, system realities, resources, accountability, and external support. This section applies the structure element of the Donabedian framework for UME and GME programs to plan and execute continuous improvement and sustainment.

Curricular Features: Time, Sequence, Changes, and Explicit Integration With Other Portions of the School Curriculum

Curricular change is a necessary, challenging, and complex part of HSS implementation in both UME and GME. Finding space for HSS content is commonly noted in the literature.[27,28] Institutions can use this chapter to develop a curriculum modification strategy to drive change within their allotted time frame and avoid getting bogged down with space challenges in the curriculum. Curricular change can include implementing HSS topics, highlighting them in existing sessions, changing current HSS sessions, or even integrating HSS with other curricular threads such as ethics, professional identity formation, and medical decision-making, to name a few. Whichever curricular change approach is used, understanding how the change will impact contact hours and communicating with the key stakeholders (e.g., curriculum committees, module directors, and course directors) is critical for HSS curriculum improvement and sustainability success. Early and frequent communication regarding the effect changes have on curriculum learning objectives, content, and faculty development sessions will build trust, confidence, and legitimacy in the HSS curriculum and its leaders.

Gaining and Building Buy-in From Faculty, Preceptors, Leadership, and Students: A Commitment to Institutional Mission and Culture and Commitment of Executive Leadership to the Curriculum

Gaining and maintaining buy-in from faculty, preceptors, leadership, and students is a cyclical and enduring process. For this reason, the HSS leadership team should consist of faculty from differing health professions and hierarchical levels within the institution and include advisory from learners. This composition allows for broad ownership, positive messaging to diverse disciplines, extended alliances, and institutional support needed for curriculum success.[29,30] Additionally, there are three categories of stakeholders that programs should consider when gaining and maintaining buy-in for HSS implementation and sustainment. These stakeholders include preceptors (clinical faculty during the clerkship phase and in GME), leadership, and learners (Table 7.1).

Additionally, many HSS educators are practitioners in health systems (e.g., director of QI, patient safety officer, or director of operations) and come from other fields such as social science.[28] These HSS educators may have little experience in the medical education environment compared with seasoned basic and clinical science faculty. Although it is impossible to control the amount of scientific discovery in HSS, the promotion of scholarly activity in HSS is highly encouraged and needed to close the gaps in knowledge. Institutions can address faculty development with their HSS educators by designing sessions focused on medical education teaching and assessment techniques.

Clinical Learning Environment

Going beyond the academic setting and into the health systems to see HSS in action may be a challenge for most

TABLE 7.1   Strategies for Successful Buy-in of Health Systems Science Curricula — By Stakeholder

Stakeholder	Challenges	Strategies for Success
Preceptors	Preceptors are hesitant to add or develop additional HSS content to their responsibilities.	Carefully consider high-quality off-the-shelf HSS curriculum items and products that can be implemented seamlessly.
Leaders	Keeping senior leadership engaged and supportive of HSS programs is cyclical and ongoing.	Schedule early and frequent curriculum updates with senior leadership; these updates build trust, buy-in, and essential lines of communication. Highlight links with accreditation.
Learners	Learners lack interest or understanding of the importance of HSS content, especially early in their training.[28]	Prime learners on the institution's commitment to and focus on HSS during the recruitment process to help recruit early HSS adopters.[28] Explicitly start each HSS session by emphasizing "how the content of this session can distinguish you" conveys the value of developing the session's HSS competency to the learner for successful doctoring.[31] Encourage faculty use a one-voice approach on sharing the relevance of HSS in GME with learners. 1. HSS is a common topic during residency matching interviews. 2. HSS is a core requirement during GME training. 3. Learning HSS during UME better prepares learners for professional success in GME.
Learners	Learners cannot relate to applying HSS knowledge and content based on their limited work experience (this can vary from learner to learner) in the health care setting.	Consider delivering HSS content in the IPE setting. These IPE sessions could include graduate-level nursing, physician assistant, or health administration learners who may have relevant experience in the health care delivery setting.
HSS educators	HSS practitioners lack of teaching experience with UME and GME learners.	Design faculty development sessions for practitioners who focus on medical education teaching and assessment techniques.

GME, Graduate medical education; *HSS,* health systems science; *IPE,* interprofessional education; *UME,* undergraduate medical education.

(if not all) HSS teams. Many clinicians are not trained on HSS competency domains. However, there are some health care professionals who have keen HSS competencies. Even though they may not speak the HSS language, they can effectively train learners in HSS competencies and demonstrate these skills in the system. More commonly, though, clinicians in the system may not model HSS competencies. Learners in their clinical rotations will likely notice this gap and question the importance of HSS skills and competencies when they do not see physicians role model HSS competencies. Planning HSS faculty development for those who serve as preceptors during clinical rotations is one way to address this incongruence in theory and practice of HSS within the health system.

Faculty Time, Faculty Development, and Technology

Resources are a significant factor in the success and sustainment of any program or curriculum. Resources for HSS improvement and sustainment must include careful attention to allocating money for faculty, staff, technology, and educational materials. HSS teams quickly realize the demand for dedicated faculty, staff, and other support during implementation, improvement, and sustainment. Creating HSS strategic goals (i.e., results related to critical success factors) is one of the best ways for medical educators to quickly see the need for various resources to achieve the goals.[32] From the strategic goals, institutions can develop a list of resources needed to achieve each goal, and from there, create an HSS budget.

Human capital will likely encompass the most significant part of an HSS budget. Defining and updating roles and responsibilities for each member of the HSS team keeps the program on track for achieving its strategic goals. Managing human capital closely and engaging in succession planning is a substantial part of HSS leadership and is a critical success factor. Ensuring that a program has subject matter experts in each of the core competency domains while continually scanning institutions and health systems for additional faculty builds resiliency. It is noteworthy that retention of HSS faculty and staff is less resource intensive than recruitment. Retention efforts can include robust research and conference funding, faculty development, and a working culture of value and respect.

Institutional Hierarchy and Reporting Relationships

Institutional hierarchy creates organization and structure in an institution. The most common form of this hierarchy is published in organizational charts. Organizational charts reflect lines of accountability and areas of responsibilities of leaders. Having HSS represented on the institution's organizational chart reflects proper structure and accountability of the HSS program. Revisiting and updating an organization's structure is a critical piece of program or curriculum sustainability and growth. Other accountability considerations include the organization's curriculum committee. Updates to and engagement with the curriculum oversight committee provide a layer of legitimacy to HSS curricula. Additionally, institutional stakeholder boards or advisory boards require attention to ensure the HSS program meets their needs. Feedback from stakeholder and advisory bodies is an integral part of the CQI process.

External Resources

Scanning and using external resources and support from professional organizations, academic institutions, and other platforms can provide excellent opportunities for HSS direction, guidance, and learning material. External resources will likely stimulate change in a program's strategic goals (both short- and long-term goals) and assist in keeping pace with changes in the field of HSS. Moreover, faculty completion of the AMA HSS Scholars program is another way to bring rigor to the HSS program at any institution.[33] This program also provides access to HSS specific resources and educational offerings. Additional resources for HSS material include the AMA HSS textbook and HSS topical materials for teaching.[34,35]

PROCESS CHALLENGES TO CONTINUOUS QUALITY IMPROVEMENT

Establishing and sustaining HSS curricula as equal to clinical and basic science curricula is fundamental to achieving HSS program goals in the long term. HSS helps the basic and clinical sciences achieve the greatest impact, particularly when making changes in a population's health and getting at the Quadruple Aim. The three-pillar model of medical education can be a true partnership through collaboration and a shared vision, which is ideally created by the institution's leadership and curriculum committee. This commitment to the three-pillar model requires a top-down and bottom-up approach when it comes to operationalizing the model. This means that the top leaders in the institution and the HSS team and instructors collectively work in their sphere of influence to use and improve systems that ensure equal partnership across HSS as well as the clinical and basic sciences.

Another way HSS programs works to deliver the desired outcome of systems citizens is coalescing multiple threads of medical education topics during HSS learning.[17] This approach serves as an opportunity to build HSS competencies in other medical education topics and for learners to realize the application of HSS topics to different contextual settings. For example, a learner's ability to recognize a value-based care dilemma during a pharmacology session builds their confidence in HSS competencies and showcases the practical use of HSS in various settings. Working with basic and clinical science faculty in building integrated sessions builds the learner's investment in HSS and demonstrates equal pillar partnership.

The final consideration in sustaining and improving HSS programs is ongoing faculty development. Annual or semiannual access to HSS faculty development sessions allows new or current faculty to learn about HSS and may encourage incremental engagement in the HSS program. Research presentations at institutions by seminal HSS scholars can provide an additional layer of legitimacy and focus toward HSS curriculum efforts.

OUTCOME CHALLENGES TO CONTINUOUS QUALITY IMPROVEMENT

The most significant part of CQI and sustainment is meaningful measurement of program outcomes. Measurement serves as the base of knowledge and data to ensure desired learning outcomes are met, and if not, it serves as the impetus for planning improvements. Although short- and long-term strategic HSS goals are pieces of the puzzle to get closer to achieving the overall HSS mission, institutions cannot forget to measure the primary desired outcomes of the HSS program. For example, one strategic goal could be to "increase interprofessional education (IPE) sessions that focus on health care structures and processes, management and advocacy, teaming, and systems thinking." Meeting this strategic goal will likely get the HSS program one step closer to reaching its ultimate mission. For example, a UME program's mission (or statement of purpose) may be "The health systems science curriculum teaches university faculty and students to be transformational leaders, problem solvers, and mission-oriented systems thinkers who are prepared to improve the health of those we serve." How institutions measure whether they are meeting the curriculum's mission matters, particularly for sustainment and CQI.

Going back to the earlier example, measuring the example institution's strategic goal to increase IPE is straightforward. It would involve measuring both the IPE sessions' evaluation of the learners or their understanding and learning of the session material and assessment or feedback from the learners on the faculties' delivery of the sessions that either aided or hindered learning. Measuring strategic goals is necessary for both the short- and long-term success of the curriculum. Demonstrating achievement of strategic goals, through measurement, fosters CQI momentum and signals to institution leadership the program's growth.

What institutions measure matters and feeds into decision-making, planning, and goal setting. Measuring outcomes versus outputs may be difficult, especially across portions of the collective curricula or program. Selecting what measurements indicate mission achievement, and then deciding how to collect the data is equally important. Establishing a systematic way to collect data may include using a curriculum management system, which is also a standard for accrediting bodies in UME.[36] Using technology to assist in measuring outcomes can decrease measurement error and easily adapt to changes in measurement (e.g., new measurement variables, drilling down on data). Additionally, as HSS curriculum owners build learners' competency in core HSS domains, curriculum leaders can track competency development touchpoints using a curriculum management system. Curriculum tracking systems are useful for identifying HSS competency development gaps and for systematically building competency proficiency levels (e.g., novice, intermediate, advanced) incrementally across the curriculum.

Assessing and understanding the results of the HSS education program are a vital part of CQI and sustainment. Through a larger lens, as institutions develop system citizens an even more significant measurement opportunity is documenting how HSS learners add value to patients and the health system. Sequentially, after measuring these outcomes, the next step is actively pursuing and managing change. Challenges to curricular improvement include failing to make changes to HSS sessions based on previous feedback because of lack of time or inertia, administrative barriers to curricular changes based on curriculum committee requirements, and lack of resources or faculty to teach identified HSS competency domain gaps (e.g., clinical informatics). Overcoming these barriers to change takes keen focus by HSS and institutional leaders applying accountability. For example, annual program reports that highlight HSS curricular goals, achievements, assessment, and improvements are one way for institutions to hold program owners accountable. A combination of oversight and leadership can break down these barriers to change.

USING CONTINUOUS QUALITY IMPROVEMENT PROCESSES TO DEVELOP SUSTAINABILITY

Achieving the long-term goals of HSS education initiatives requires educators to continuously ensure ongoing progress toward the explicit HSS program or curricular goals. At the broadest level and as previously mentioned, HSS content in UME or GME should be evaluated as a part of the HSS committee or curriculum committee. Much like the systematic review of other UME (e.g., basic science blocks, clerkships) and GME (rotation) content, the HSS curriculum or program review should include an evaluation on currency, relevancy, integration, and goal attainment. Faculty and learner feedback can be used to ensure HSS topics align with clinical materials and experiences by week, month, and block or rotation. An annual review ensures that as the overall UME curriculum or GME program changes, integration with HSS content remains. Sustaining HSS programs requires continuous monitoring at the broadest level. Using the curriculum committee has the added benefit that faculty and learner stakeholders are involved in the process, aware of the content, and informed of any changes. It also ensures accreditation bodies (Liaison Committee on Medical Education or LCME; ACGME) are aware of the HSS program and its importance in a school or program's overall medical education. Educators must also address other factors for success, such as ongoing faculty development (for those teaching in the formal curriculum and front-line clinicians who deliver bedside clinical teaching) and a conducive clinical learning environment.

Continuous quality improvement of the explicit or formal curriculum includes constant monitoring of curricular integration, content, and delivery as well as learner outcomes as described in logic models. Deming's **plan, do, study, act (PDSA)** loop (Fig. 7.2) for CQI as described in the Institute for Healthcare Improvement's Model for Improvement and in Chapter 3 can be used to assess an HSS curriculum at multiple levels.[37,38] In this context, the PDSA cycle starts with *planning* an HSS curriculum followed by *do*, which includes the implementation of an improved feature of practice. The third phase requires the *study* of the outcomes articulated in the logic model to determine whether they lead to the desired changes. This includes a review of the content, design, and integration of the HSS curriculum. Based on the results of the study phase, opportunities for improvement should be identified. During the *act* phase, educators work with a team to adjust the goals, change the content, or modify curricular integration. The four steps of the cycle provide the best outcomes when they are repeated as part of the CQI and sustainability process and developed across all levels of the HSS curriculum.

Deming's vision was to use PDSA cycles as part of CQI. Although an HSS team may feel a great deal of satisfaction after they have planned and implemented a curriculum, that is only the beginning. Just as medical knowledge changes, so does HSS knowledge. Sustaining the relevancy and integration of the HSS curriculum is an ongoing process. It requires a team of dedicated faculty who are committed to improving the content, delivery, and integration of the program. It requires work, but the payoff is tremendous—a new generation of physicians who can integrate basic science, clinical science, and HSS to optimize the Quadruple Aim.

One of the benefits of applying the PDSA cycle in HSS curricula is that it provides a framework for assessing the relevancy and coverage of the HSS curriculum topic areas. For example, if an HSS curriculum has patient safety as a topic area, the faculty responsible for this content can use the PDSA cycle to ensure the lectures and activities within this topic area collectively meet the expected goals. Using PDSA at this level in the HSS curriculum may show opportunities for improvement caused by coverage gaps or content overlap. Faculty leaders may also identify needed changes in where and how the materials are integrated into the clinical topics. Obtaining stakeholder input is critical to determining if the materials are presented in the best sequence and at the right time in the overall medical education. As the HSS curriculum matures, it is necessary to monitor the curriculum at the topical level.

Improving the HSS content requires continuous monitoring at the lecture and activity level. PDSA cycles can be used by the content expert to improve the delivery of the materials. Inputs such as learner assessments and evaluations are good resources to study the attainment of expected outcomes. Learners may provide insight into how the materials could be improved in presentation, relevancy, and integration. Feedback on didactic and experiential activities and faculty facilitation of learning can be readily used to make rapid improvements in the HSS curriculum.

CONCLUSION

There is no one-size-fits-all approach to sustainability, and this chapter does not include all theories of long-term sustainability in every HSS teaching and learning context. Although this chapter provides the foundational theories for sustainability and its key elements of evaluating and improving HSS programs, the application of these principles can be modified and adjusted to fit institutional needs. Indeed, a vital feature of an institution's ability to sustain change over time is its ability to recognize when a specific approach to sustainability is not working and swiftly change course. Learning organizations employ modifications when they discover new information, and this dynamic approach to sustainability ultimately serves as the aspirational goal for HSS curriculum leaders and faculty.

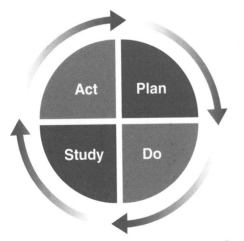

Fig. 7.2 Deming's plan, do, study, act cycle. (From Deming, W. Edwards. The PDSA cycle. In: The New Economics for Industry, Government, Education. 3rd ed. Cambridge: Massachusetts Institute of Technology; 91.)

TAKE-HOME POINTS

1. Long-term sustainability for HSS education programs is a dynamic process of adapting to new and evolving demands.
2. Selection of an overarching planning framework and evidenced-based models of sustainability, such as Kotter's process of change management and the PSAT, can guide program developers to collect relevant macro- and meso-level data that can be used to respond to challenges and barriers as they arise.
3. At the micro level of planning, logic models enable teams to map the implementation process and guide

steps in operationalizing the macro-level strategic plan.
4. Logic models help identify misalignments between outcomes, outputs, activities, and resources and highlight necessary changes for CQI.
5. In addition to selecting appropriate planning and mapping frameworks to support sustainability, it is important to use well-tested evaluation and CQI paradigms such as Kirkpatrick's evaluation model; Donabedian's structure, process, and outcomes model; and Deming's PDSA loop.

QUESTIONS FOR FURTHER THOUGHT

1. Does your HSS program have a logic model? How can faculty and stakeholders use the logic model to measure success and to identify improvement opportunities?
2. When it comes to your HSS program, what are the key barriers to gaining and building buy-in from faculty,

preceptors, and leadership? What strategies can you use to overcome these barriers?
3. How can you establish reliable and effective budget and administrative support to secure resources for sustaining your program over the long-term?

VIGNETTE 1

It has been 6 years since the Alta Dena School of Medicine has implemented its new health systems science (HSS) curriculum. With support from the dean, the associate deans of preclinical and clinical curricula, and a host of excited faculty, the longitudinal program has been popular with each successive class of students. Now senior administrators are beginning to ask: Does the program make a difference to our students and the programs they serve?

Tasked with examining this question, a team from the Office of Medical Education Research begins to assemble the data they have collected on the program since its first year. However, they quickly find substantial gaps between the program's stated goals and the kinds of data collected. Most courses included end of course student satisfaction surveys, but few data sources could attest to whether the program met its learning outcomes, behavioral objectives, or impact goals.

As a result, the team could not make any specific claims or recommendations about the efficacy of the school's HSS curriculum. Furthermore, the evaluation team has no systematic way to collect data from graduates of the program in residency, making it difficult to assess the program's long-term impact. Without the right data, senior administrators are starting to wonder whether the curricular time spent on the HSS program is worth the trouble after all.

Thought Questions
1. How might a logic model have helped to support the development of a more comprehensive program evaluation process?
2. In what ways could a direct pathway from inputs to outcomes have helped to support the sustainability of the program in the long term?

VIGNETTE 2

Administrators at a large academic medical center have enlisted a group of residents to help develop a new module on systems citizenship that would be offered to a special interest group at the hospital that includes medical students, residents, and attending physicians. As part of the design process, the residents have

reviewed the literature; summarized key features of the concept; and developed a short presentation for the students, their fellow residents, and attendings. However, they soon arrive at a stumbling block: How will they assess the success of their module? Some residents suggest creating a simple multiple-choice test to check individuals' knowledge about the core content, but others suggest this is too simplistic. Another group of residents suggests creating a self-diagnostic checklist to help attendees gauge their own competence as systems citizens, but others argue most attendees would not faithfully complete self-diagnostics. As they discuss this challenge, the residents come to an impasse.

Thought Questions

1. How might they assess their learners' knowledge and enactment of such a complex HSS concept?
2. What kind of overall learner assessment strategy might you suggest to the residents?

ANNOTATED BIBLIOGRAPHY

Gonzalo JD, Baxley E, Borkan J, et al. Priority areas and potential solutions for successful integration and sustainment of health systems science in undergraduate medical education. *Acad Med.* 2017;92(1):63-69.

This study uses 2 years of data collected from a working group of 11 American Medical Association Accelerating Change in Medical Education Consortium programs, all initiating and implementing health systems science (HSS) curricula. Thematic content analysis and constant comparative analyses point to curriculum implementation challenges. Additionally, the authors lay out several priority areas and potential solutions to overcome HSS implementation challenges and advance HSS. Developing comprehensive, standardized, and integrated curriculum and assessment are possible solutions to advancing HSS and enhancing HSS teachers' knowledge and skills.

Lennox L, Maher L, Reed J. Navigating the sustainability landscape: a systematic review of sustainability approaches in healthcare. *Implement Sci.* 2018;13(1):27.

In this systematic review of program sustainability approaches in health care, the authors identify 62 publications that evaluated a sustainability approach, representing a large range of frameworks, models, and tools. Despite the heterogeneity of approaches and studies, the authors identified six key constructs that were essential to measure across the initiatives: (1) initiative design and delivery, (2) negotiating iterative processes, (3) people involved, (4) resources, (5) the organizational setting, and (6) the external environment. Although not every study reported on each construct, these six features of sustainability appeared in 75% of the total published studies in the review. Efforts in HSS education would benefit from considering these six features of sustainability during planning, design, implementation, and evaluation of new programs to ensure that key issues of sustainability are integrated from the outset.

Ridinger HA, Bonnet K, Schlundt DG, Tekian A, Riddle J, Lomis KD. Defining successful practice within health systems science among entering residents: a single-institution qualitative study of graduate medical education faculty observations. *Acad Med.* 2021;96(11S):S126-S135.

The authors conducted 17 semistructured qualitative interviews of graduate medical education faculty leaders at Vanderbilt University Medical Center. After coding, data were aligned with a logic model for HSS-prepared entering residents. Faculty further describe domain-specific knowledge and skills. The logic model is an excellent depiction of how this framework can inform curricula development, evaluation, and improvement to ensure students learn and demonstrate the expected competencies.

Sklar DP. Implementing curriculum change. *Acad Med.* 2018; 93(10):1417-1419.

This article discusses key considerations when revising curricula so that valuable changes can be sustained over time. It discusses two approaches to curriculum change, either through a narrower track approach, which may be easier to initiate, or through global change for more substantive topics. The article notes that it is imperative to align curricular and health systems goals and provide meaningful opportunities for student input, as well as that curriculum change needs to be thought of in the context of clinical care environments. Curriculum design and assessment must be tightly coupled to ensure student learning and to provide evaluation data to contribute to program sustainment.

REFERENCES

1. Bodkin A, Hakimi S. Sustainable by design: a systematic review of factors for health promotion program sustainability. *BMC Public Health.* 2020;20(1):964-980.
2. Shelton RC, Cooper BR, Stirman SW. The sustainability of evidence-based interventions and practices in public health and Health Care. *Annu Rev Public Health.* 2018;39(1):55-76.
3. Kotter JP. *Leading Change.* Boston: Harvard Business Review Press; 2012.
4. Schell SF, Luke DA, Schooley MW, et al. Public health program capacity for sustainability: a new framework. *Implement Sci.* 2013;8:15-24.
5. Moullin JC, Sabater-Hernández D, Fernandez-Llimos F, Benrimoj SI. A systematic review of implementation frameworks of innovations in healthcare and resulting generic implementation framework. *Health Res Policy Syst.* 2015;13:16-27.
6. Harrison R, Fischer S, Walpola RL, et al. Where do models for change management, improvement and implementation meet? A systematic review of the applications of change management models in healthcare. *J Healthc Leadersh.* 2021;13: 85-108.
7. Luke DA, Calhoun A, Robichaux CB, Elliott MB, Moreland-Russell S. The program sustainability assessment tool: a new instrument for public health programs. *Prev Chronic Dis.* 2014;11:130184.
8. Calhoun A, Mainor A, Moreland-Russell S, Maier RC, Brossart L, Luke DA. Using the program sustainability assessment tool to assess and plan for sustainability. *Prev Chronic Dis.* 2014;11:130185.

9. Irwin C, Strambler M, Meyer J. *The Value of Logic Models in Education*. <https://medicine.yale.edu/news-article/the-value-of-logic-models-in-education>; 2017. Accessed 18.04.22.

10. Shakman K, Rodriguez S. *Logic Models for Program Design, Implementation, and Evaluation: Workshop Toolkit*. <https://ies.ed.gov/ncee/edlabs/regions/northeast/pdf/REL_2015057.pdf>; 2015. Accessed 18.04.22.

11. Ridinger HA, Bonnet K, Schlundt DG, Tekian A, Riddle J, Lomis KD. Defining successful practice within health systems science among entering residents: a single-institution qualitative study of graduate medical education faculty observations. *Acad Med*. 2021;96(11S):S126-S135.

12. Kirkpatrick JD, Kirkpatrick WK. *Kirkpatrick's Four Levels of Training Evaluation*. Association for Talent Development; Alexandria, VA, 2016.

13. Linfield K, Posavac E. *Program Evaluation: Methods and Case Studies*. New York, NY Routledge; 2019.

14. Mengel F, Sauermann J, Zölitz U. Gender bias in teaching evaluations. *J Eur Econ Assoc*. 2019;17(2):535-566.

15. Bassett J, Cleveland A, Acorn D, Nix M, Snyder T. Are they paying attention? Students' lack of motivation and attention potentially threaten the utility of course evaluations. *Assess Eval High Educ*. 2017;42(3):431-442.

16. Deslauriers L, McCarty LS, Miller K, Callaghan K, Kestin G. Measuring actual learning versus feeling of learning in response to being actively engaged in the classroom. *Proc Natl Acad Sci*. 2019;116(39):19251-19257.

17. Gonzalo JD, Davis C, Thompson BM, Haidet P. Unpacking medical students' mixed engagement in health systems science education. *Teach Learn Med*. 2020;32(3):250-258.

18. Gonzalo JD, Baxley E, Borkan J, et al. Priority areas and potential solutions for successful integration and sustainment of health systems science in undergraduate medical education. *Acad Med*. 2017;92(1):63-69.

19. Gonzalo JD, Chang A, Dekhtyar M, Starr SR, Holmboe E, Wolpaw DR. Health systems science in medical education: unifying the components to catalyze transformation. *Acad Med*. 2020;95(9):1362-1372.

20. Davis CR, Gonzalo JD. How medical schools can promote community collaboration through health systems science education? *AMA J Ethics*. 2019;21(3):E239-E247.

21. Donabedian A. The quality of care: how can it be assessed? *JAMA*. 1988;260(12):1743-1748.

22. Botma Y, Labuschagne M. Application of the Donabedian quality assurance approach in developing an educational programme. *Innov Educ Teach Int*. 2019;56(3):363-372.

23. Bodenheimer T, Sinsky C. From triple to quadruple aim: care of the patient requires care of the provider. *Ann Fam Med*. 2014;12(6):573-576.

24. Scheirer MA. Is sustainability possible? A review and commentary on empirical studies of program sustainability. *Am J Eval*. 2005;26(3):320-347.

25. Lennox L, Maher L, Reed J. Navigating the sustainability landscape: a systematic review of sustainability approaches in healthcare. *Implement Sci*. 2018;13(1):27-44.

26. LoPorto J. Application of the Donabedian quality-of-care model to New York State Direct Support Professional Core Competencies: how Structure, process, and outcomes impacts disability services. *J Soc Change*. 2020;12(1):40-70.

27. Sklar DP. Implementing curriculum change. *Acad Med*. 2018;93(10):1417-1419.

28. Gonzalo JD, Ogrinc G. Health systems science: the "broccoli" of undergraduate medical education. *Acad Med*. 2019;94(10):1425-1432.

29. Borkan JM, George P, Tunkel AR. Curricular transformation. *Acad Med*. 2018;93(10):1428-1430.

30. Novak DA, Hallowell R, Ben-Ari R, Elliott D. A continuum of innovation: curricular renewal strategies in undergraduate medical education, 2010-2018. *Acad Med*. 2019;94(11S):S79-S85.

31. Borkan JM, Hammoud MM, Nelson E, et al. Health systems science education: the new post-Flexner professionalism for the 21st century. *Med Teach*. 2021;43(suppl 2):S25-S31.

32. Ginter PM, Duncan WJ, Swayne LE. *Strategic Management of Healthcare Organizations*. Hoboken, NJ: Wiley; 2018.

33. American Medical Association. *Health Systems Science Scholars*. <https://www.ama-assn.org/education/accelerating-change-medical-education/health-systems-science-scholars>; Accessed 18.04.22.

34. Skochelak SE, Hammoud MM, Lomis KD. *Health Systems Science*. St. Louis: Elsevier; 2021.

35. American Medical Association. *AMA Health Systems Science Leaning Series*. <https://edhub.ama-assn.org/health-systems-science>; 2022. Accessed 18.04.22.

36. Changiz T, Yamani N, Tofighi S, Zoubin F, Eghbali B. Curriculum management/monitoring in undergraduate medical education: a systematized review. *BMC Med Educ*. 2019;19(1):60-69.

37. Institute for Healthcare Improvement. *Science of Improvement: Testing Changes*. <http://www.ihi.org/resources/Pages/HowtoImprove/ScienceofImprovementTestingChanges.aspx>; Accessed 18.04.22.

38. Taylor MJ, McNicholas C, Nicolay C, Darzi A, Bell D, Reed E. Systematic review of the application of the plan–do–study–act method to improve quality in healthcare. *BMJ Qual Saf*. 2014;23(4):290-298.

active learning An approach to instruction that involves actively engaging students with the course material through discussions, problem solving, case studies, role plays, and other methods.

assets The tools and resources an organization can use to implement change.

Association of American Medical Colleges A nonprofit association dedicated to transforming health through medical education, health care, medical research, and community collaborations.

asynchronous learning Teaching and learning occur at different times. This allows students to learn on their own schedules within a certain timeframe by accessing and completing online lectures, readings, homework, and other learning materials at any time.

balancing measures Determine whether changes designed to improve one part of the system are causing new problems in other parts of the system.

Bloom's Taxonomy A hierarchical model used to classify educational learning objectives into levels of complexity and specificity.

change concept A general notion or approach to change that has been found to be useful in developing specific ideas for changes that lead to improvement.

change management The methods and manners in which an organization describes and implements change within both its internal and external processes.

clinical decision support (CDS) A component of health information technology that provides clinicians, staff, patients, or other individuals knowledge and person-specific information, intelligently filtered or presented at appropriate times, to enhance health and health care. CDS tools include computerized alerts and reminders to physicians, other care providers, and patients; clinical guidelines; condition-specific order sets; focused patient data reports and summaries; documentation templates; diagnostic support; and contextually relevant reference information, among other tools.

clinical learning environment Anywhere students (and other learners) are engaged in patient care for the purpose of their own learning.

collaborative examinations A method in which students work together to complete a written evaluative exam.

continuous quality improvement (CQI) A deliberate, defined, ongoing process focused on improving health care delivery.

Core Entrustable Professional Activities for Entering Residency (CEPAER) Activities defined by the Association of American Medical Colleges that residents should be able to perform on the first day of residency without direct supervision, regardless of specialty choice.

driver diagram A visual display of a team's theory of what contributes to the achievement of a project aim.

early adopters Faculty and students who integrate concept(s) early in the implementation process and who can serve as exemplary champions of the concept(s).

failure mode and effect analysis The process of reviewing as many components, assemblies, and subsystems as possible to identify potential failure modes in a system and their causes and effects.

formal curricula Classroom-based learning, or for graduate medical education, outside a patient encounter. This curriculum addresses cognitive objectives such as learning nomenclature and includes lectures, small group discussions, and problem-solving exercises.

health care inequities Avoidable differences in health care received by different groups of people.

health systems science (HSS) A foundational platform and framework for the study and understanding of how care is delivered, how health professionals work together to deliver this care, and how the health system can improve patient care and health care delivery.

health systems science (HSS) core domains These include health system improvement; value in health care; population, public, and social determinants of health; clinical informatics and health technology; health care policy and economics; and health care process and structure.

hidden curricula Unwritten, unofficial, and often unintended lessons, values, and perspectives that students learn in school.

high-reliability team A group of people gathered to manage a high-risk situation with a high degree of effectiveness.

implementation science The scientific study of methods and strategies that facilitate the uptake of evidence-based practice and research into regular use by practitioners and policymakers.

informal curricula Education that can occur outside of a structured curriculum.

intercollaborative practice When multiple health workers from different professional backgrounds work together with patients, families, caregivers, and communities to deliver the highest quality of care across settings.

Interprofessional Education Collaborative (IPEC) A group consisting of the Association of American Medical Colleges and five other health care organizations involved with the formalized education of their profession, including nursing, pharmacy, public health, osteopathic medicine, and dentistry.

interprofessional practice When multiple physicians and other health care professionals from different disciplines and specialties work together with patients, families, caregivers, and communities to deliver the highest quality of care.

Kirkpatrick's training evaluation model A globally recognized method of evaluating the results of training and learning programs. It has four levels: reaction, learning, behavior, and results.

Liaison Committee on Medical Education Accrediting body for educational programs at schools of medicine in the United States and Canada.

logic model A program planning tool to help with program design.

master adaptive learner   A learner who uses a metacognitive approach to self-regulated learning that leads to the development and demonstration of adaptive expertise.

medical education program objectives   The skills, attitudes, and knowledge that graduating medical students should possess.

Miller's pyramid   A figure to help faculty and educational program leaders understand the progressive and developmental acquisition of clinical competence and how different assessment tools may be applied.

narrative assessments   The analysis of a story told by an individual to assess language and communication or written evaluations of the clinical performance of a learner.

objective structured clinical examination (OSCE)   Hands-on examinations designed to test competence in skills such as communication, clinical examination, medical procedures and prescription, and other skills required for clinical practice, frequently through the use of simulation sessions and engagement with standardized patients.

outcomes   Effects on patients and populations, including knowledge and behaviors.

outcome measures   Measures chosen to assess the impact of implementing a health systems science curriculum.

passive learning   Method of learning or instruction where students receive information from the instructor and internalize it. The learner receives no feedback from the instructor.

plan, do, study, act (PDSA) cycle   Part of the Institute for Healthcare Improvement's Model for Improvement. Steps in the PDSA cycle are Step 1: Plan—Plan the test or observation, including a plan for collecting data. Step 2: Do—Try out the test. Step 3: Study—Set aside time to analyze the data and study the results. Step 4: Act—Refine the change based on what was learned from the test.

pre-clerkship   The first part of medical school, frequently predominantly didactic. Medical students learn basic sciences.

pre-implementation   The initial phase of curriculum implementation that permits a more holistic view of the challenges and requirements of curriculum implementation and identifies targeted strategies that address potential challenges at the onset of curriculum change.

problem-based learning   A student-centered approach in which students learn about a subject by working in groups to solve an open-ended problem and create their own learning objectives.

process measures   Assesses whether the parts or steps in the system are performing as planned.

processes   The activities or steps in performing routine work in caring for patients.

professional identity formation   A complex and transformational process of internalizing a profession's core values and beliefs.

program evaluation   A systematic method for collecting, analyzing, and using information to answer questions about projects, policies, and programs, particularly about their effectiveness and efficiency.

psychological safety   When someone feels safe to authentically share their values, experiences, perspectives, and concerns and feels safe to explore difficult topics such as feedback, conflicts, or equity and belonging issues.

Quadruple Aim   Includes the three aspects of the Triple Aim (improving the patient experience of care, improving the health of populations, and reducing the per capita cost of health care) with the addition of health care professional wellness.

scale   To increase the size of a health systems science curriculum.

spread   To expand a health systems science curriculum beyond the initial department.

stakeholders   Those who are implementing a health systems science curriculum, or who will be affected by its implementation.

SWOT analysis   A strategic planning technique used to help a person or organization identify strengths, weaknesses, opportunities, and threats.

systems citizen   Any health care professional who uses systems-thinking skills in their professional role to contribute to the holistic needs of individual patients, populations, and the health system itself.

systems thinking   Recognizing and understanding the complex interdependencies and relationships within a functional system such as health care. Allows the formation of linkages among disparate areas of activity in health care to improve outcomes, patient experience, and value in health care.

simulation   A teaching method that tests participants' knowledge and skill levels by placing them in scenarios in which they must actively solve problems.

SMART goals   An acronym that stands for specific, measurable, achievable, relevant, and time based.

spiral learning   A teaching method based on the premise that a student learns more about a subject each time the topic is reviewed or encountered.

structural measures   Assess features of a health care organization or clinic relevant to capacity to provide health care.

structures   The resources (e.g., people, equipment, supplies) required to complete the clinical activities or process steps to achieve the desired clinical outcomes.

sustainability   The ability to be maintained at a certain rate or level.

systems-based practice   Actions that demonstrate an awareness of and responsiveness to the larger context and system of health care, and the ability to call on system resources effectively to provide care that is of optimal value.

systems thinking   Recognizes and understands the complex interdependencies and relationships within a functional system such as health care. Allows the formation of linkages among disparate areas of activity in health care to improve outcomes, patient experience, and value in health care.

team science   An understanding of teams, their structures, and critical elements.

Triple Aim   A framework developed by the Institute for Healthcare Improvement describing an approach to optimizing health system performance. It includes improving the patient experience of care (including quality and satisfaction), improving the health of populations, and reducing the per capita cost of health care.

value-added roles   Designed to provide students with opportunities to engage in health systems science and clinical skills while adding value to the health care system by legitimately contributing to patient care. Alternate definition: Experiential roles for students in practice environments that have the potential to positively impact individual patient and population health outcomes, costs of care, or other processes within the health system while also enhancing student knowledge, attitudes, and skills in the clinical or health systems sciences.

value stream mapping A lean tool that uses a flowchart documenting every step in the process.

INDEX

Page numbers followed by '*f*' indicate figures those followed by '*t*' indicate tables and '*b*' indicate boxes.

A

AAMC. *See* Association of American Medical College (AAMC)
Accreditation Council for Graduate Medical Education (ACGME), 3, 20, 109
Accreditation Council for Graduate Medical Education (ACGME) Milestones 2.0, 66, 80, 80–81t
Active learning, 42
Activities logic model, 106
Adult learning, optimization, 41, 42t
Advanced learners, 86, 87b
Advancing Health Equity in Clinical Practice, 61
Alliance for Academic Internal Medicine, 20
American College of Physicians, 20
American Medical Association (AMA), 3, 109
  Accelerating Change in Medical Education Consortium's HSS competency workgroup, 19, 20
  Health Systems Science Learning Series, 44
  Master Adaptive Learner, 36
Assessment for Collaborative Environments (ACE-15), 93
Assessment of Interprofessional Team Collaboration Scale (AITCS), 93
Assets, 2, 5, 15
Association of American Medical College (AAMC), 86, 109
  Curriculum Inventory Report, 2
  Graduation Questionnaire, 20
Asynchronous learning, 41
Attitude-specific assessment tools, 92
Attitudes Toward Health Care Teams Scale (ATHCT), 92

B

Balancing measures, 44–45
Beginning learners, 87b
Blended learning faculty development, 68, 69f
Bloom's Taxonomy, 38, 39f, 40t, 53–54
Buy-in of health systems science curricula, 111, 112t

C

Cancer Health Disparities, 61
Centers for Disease Control and Prevention (CDC), 6

Change management, 2, 4, 35, 36, 104
Chronic kidney disease (CKD), 38, 40, 40t
CKD-EPI calculation, 38
CLE. *See* Clinical learning environment (CLE)
CLER. *See* Clinical Learning Environment Review (CLER)
Clinical clerkships, educational opportunities for, 54–56, 55–56t
Clinical decision support (CDS), 53
Clinical informatics and technology, 27–30t
Clinical learning environment (CLE)
  advanced clinical integration, opportunities for, 58–61
  advanced learning opportunities, 61–62
  challenges, 62–63
  clinical clerkships, educational opportunities for, 54–56, 55–56t
  continuous quality improvement (CQI), 112
  early implementation, 52–54
    content, 53
    educational modality, 54
    learners, 53
    specific CLE, 53
    time and sequence of training, 53–54
  HSS integration, practical considerations for, 56–57
  learner and program evaluation, 62
Clinical Learning Environment Review (CLER), 3, 66, 79–80, 80–81t
CME. *See* Continuing medical education (CME)
Collaborative examinations, 40
Communication Assessment Tool-Team (CAT-T), 93
Competency
  across continuum, 21
  characteristics, 26b
  core domains, 20, 27–30t
  definition, 20
  Dreyfus model of expertise development, 21, 26t
  recommendations and accreditation standards
    GME, 22–23t
    UME, 22–23t
  subcompetency, 27–30t
  systems-based practice (SBP), 20
  systems thinking, 21

Competent learners, 86, 87b
Congestive heart failure (CHF), 58
Content mapping, 44
Continuing medical education (CME), 1, 2, 19, 99
Continuous quality improvement (CQI), 104
  clinical learning environment, 112
  curriculum change, 111
  gaining and building buy-in from faculty, preceptors, leadership, and students, 112–113
  outcome challenges, 113–114
  process challenges, 113
  structural challenges
    external resources, 113
    faculty time, faculty development, and technology, 112–113
    institutional hierarchy and reporting relationships, 113
  sustainability development, 114–115
Co-production, 7
Core domains, 2, 3, 4f, 70–71
  competency, 20, 27–30t
  current state inventory, 15, 15t
  health systems science (HSS), 2, 3, 4f
Core team, 12, 13–14t
COVID-19 pandemic, 2, 97
CQI. *See* Continuous quality improvement (CQI)
Curricular transformation, 2
Curriculum, defined, 36
Curriculum development, 2, 4
  barriers, 72
  Kern's six-step approach, 36, 86
  pre-clerkship, 36–40
  pre-implementation, 2
  professional identity formation, 36, 37–38b
Curriculum management system, 114
Curriculum tracking systems, 114

D

Distinction tracks, 78
Donabedian's framework, 44, 110–111
Dreyfus model of expertise development, 21, 26t
Driver diagram, 43

E

Early adopters, 7, 46, 68, 69
Edinburgh Postpartum Depression
  Screenings, 60–61
Educator competency, 14
Effective teamwork, 8, 9–11t, 12
Electronic health record (EHR), 53
Emergency department (ED), 53
Emergency medicine, 55–56t
Entrustable professional activities
  (EPAs), 62

F

Failure mode and effect analysis, 43
Family medicine, 55–56t
Formal curricula, 77
Foundations of Health Systems Science
  Clinical Clerkship Correlation
  Course, 60
Frontiers in Primary Care and Health
  Systems Science elective, 61

G

Gaming science innovations, 44b
Graduate medical education (GME), 3, 7,
  15, 86
  competency recommendations and
    accreditation standards, 22–23t
  HSS implementation in
    ACGME core competencies
      framework, 80, 80–81t
    ACGME requirements, 67
    alignment with health system
      organizational goals, 68
    alignment with institutional mission to
      support learning, 68
    barriers, 68
    blended learning faculty development,
      68, 69f
    challenges, 66–67
    Clinical Learning Environment Review
      (CLER), 79–80, 80–81t
    creating buy-in and value with faculty,
      68–72
    educational and development
      opportunities, 70–72
    educators, evaluation of, 82
    faculty and infrastructural resource
      needs identification, 69–70
    general needs assessment for faculty, 70t
    high-value care curricula gap analysis,
      75t, 76t
    Kern's six-step approach, 73, 73–74b,
      74–79
    patient health outcomes, 82
    return-on-investment opportunities, 67

Graduate medical education (GME)
  (Continued)
    strategies and approaches for faculty
      development, 72
    trainees as change agents, 67
Gynecology, 55–56t

H

Harvard Business Review, 86
Health care, 3, 19
  delivery, 27–30t
  inequities, 42
Healthcare Team Vitality Instrument
  (HTVI), 93
Health Policy and Systems (HPS), 61
Health system improvement, 27–30t
Health systems science (HSS), 1, 3–4
  change management, 2, 4
  core domains, 2, 3, 4f
  core team, 12, 13–14t
  current state inventory of core domains,
    15, 15t
  curricular structure, 14–15
  curriculum development, 2, 4
  educator competency, 14
  effective teamwork, 8, 9–11t, 12
  gaming science innovations, 44b
  guiding coalition, 5–7
  highly effective teams, 8
  ideal team composition, 8
  learning environment, 15
  pre-implementation, 1, 2, 7, 16
  sense of urgency, 5
  shared vision and strategy, 7–8
  systems thinking, 12
  team effectiveness, 12
  team members, 11–12
  team science, 12
Hidden curricula, 78, 79
High-reliability team, 8
High-value care (HVC) curricula, 77
High-value care (HVC) curricula gap
  analysis, 75t, 76t

I

Implementation science, 36
Individual Teamwork Observation and
  Feedback Tool (iTOFT), 93
Informal curricula, 77–78
Innovation
  adopters, 7, 7f
  gaming science, 44b
Institute of Medicine, 20
Institutional hierarchy, 113
Intercollaborative practice, 86
Internal medicine, 53, 54, 55–56t
Interprofessional Attitudes Scale (IPAS), 92

Interprofessional Collaborative Competencies
  Attainment Survey (ICCAS), 93
Interprofessional Collection, 88–89
Interprofessional education (IPE), 20, 85,
  86, 113–114
  assessment tools, 90–92t
  curricular content by learner level, 87b
  implementation
    evaluation and feedback, 89
    learning goals and objectives, 87–88
    needs assessment, 86–87
    organizational and educational
      strategies, 88–89
    problem identification, 86
  innovations, 97–99
  practical considerations, 93–94
  preclinical and clinical curricular
    activities at Johns Hopkins School
    of Medicine, 95t
  virtual platforms, 97, 98f
Interprofessional Education Collaborative
  (IPEC), 20, 86, 88–89
Interprofessional practice, 92, 94
Interprofessional Socialization and Valuing
  Scale (ISVSA-21), 93
IPE. *See* Interprofessional education (IPE)
IPEC. *See* Interprofessional Education
  Collaborative (IPEC)
IPEC Competency Self-Assessment Tool,
  92–93

K

Kern's six-step approach, 2, 3f, 73, 73–74b,
  74–79
Kirkpatrick's training evaluation model, 38,
  39f, 44, 45t, 107–110
Kotter change management model, 2, 3f, 35,
  36, 104–105

L

LCME. *See* Liaison Committee on Medical
  Education (LCME)
Learning, 113
  active, 42
  adult, 41, 42t
  asynchronous, 41
  collaborative, 42–43
  passive, 41, 43
  problem-based, 42
  self-directed, 41–42
  spiral, 93
  transformational, 40
Learning health system, 7
Liaison Committee on Medical Education
  (LCME), 20, 63, 89
Logic model, 45, 46t, 58, 59f, 106–107, 108f
Logic Model Workshop Toolkit, 106

M

Master adaptive learners, 36
MedBiquitous Curriculum Inventory
    Standardized Vocabulary
    Subcommittee, 40
Medical education program objectives
    (MEPOs), 53
Medicine as a Profession (MAP), 60
Miller's pyramid, 38, 39, 39f, 40, 41t
Multidisciplinary error analysis, 43

N

Narrative assessments, 40
National Board of Medical Examiners
    (NBME), 40, 66, 92
National Center for Interprofessional
    Practice and Education, 89
NextGen curriculum, 60

O

Objective structured clinical examinations
    (OSCEs), 40, 107
Obstetrics, 55–56t
One-size-fits-all approach, 79
Organizational assets, 2, 5
Outcome measures, 44
Outcomes, 110
Outcomes-approach logic model, 106

P

Passive learning, 41, 43
Patient Protection and Affordable Care Act,
    68, 86
Patient safety (PS), 20
Patients Insights and Views Observing
    Teams Questionnaire (PIVOT), 93
PDSA. See Plan, do, study, act (PDSA) cycle
Pediatrics, 55–56t
Physician centrality, 92
Plan, do, study, act (PDSA) cycle, 35,
    115, 115f
Policy and economics, 27–30t
Population and public health, 27–30t
Population Health Leadership, 61
Pre-clerkship curriculum
    active learning, 42
    approach, 36
    challenges, 46
    collaborative learning, 42–43
    development, 36–40
    evaluation, 44–46
    existing conditions of HSS curriculum,
        36, 37f
    integration and implementation, 43
    organizational and educational strategies,
        41–43

Pre-clerkship curriculum (Continued)
    self-directed learning, 41–42
    six-step approach, 36, 37–38b
Pre-implementation, 1, 2, 7, 16
Problem-based learning, 42
Processes, 110
Process measures, 44
Professional identity formation, 36, 37–38b,
    79, 98, 109
Program drift, 104
Program evaluation, 105
    for effectiveness and cultural change,
        107–110
    Kirkpatrick model, 107–110
    logic model, 106–107, 108f
Program Sustainability Assessment Tool
    (PSAT), 104, 105, 105b
Psychiatry, 55–56t
Psychological safety, 12, 43

Q

Quadruple Aim, 20, 66, 86, 111, 113
Quality improvement (QI), 20, 106
Quality improvement and patient safety
    (QIPS), 3

R

Recommendations
    Association of American Medical College
        (AAMC), 20
    Clinical Learning Environment Review
        (CLER), 66, 67, 79
    competency, 22–23t
Return-on-investment, 67

S

SBP. See Systems-based practice (SBP)
Scale, 4
Scholarly Inquiry (SI) Program, 61
Schools of medicine (SOM), 94
Schools of nursing (SON), 94
Schools of pharmacy (SOP), 94
Schools of public health (SPH), 94
SDH. See Social determinants of health (SDH)
Self-directed learning, 41–42
Simulation, 43, 54
SOAP (subjective, objective, assessment,
    and plan), 40
Social determinants of health (SDH), 20, 54
Specific, measurable, achievable, relevant,
    and time-based (SMART), 16
Spiral learning, 93
Stakeholders, 2, 5
    analysis, 6, 6t
    engagement, 6, 6t
    preceptors faculty, 111
    readiness, 6, 7

Story Slams, 78
Structural measures, 45
Student Perceptions of Physician-
    Pharmacist Interprofessional Clinical
    Education (SPICE-2) tool, 92
Students Perceptions of Interprofessional
    Clinical Education Revised
    (SPICE-R), 92
Subcompetency, 27–30t
Surgery, 55–56t
Sustainability, 104
    development using CQI, 114–115
    as dynamic process, 104
    planning with Kotter's model of change,
        104–105
    program evaluation, 105
        for effectiveness and cultural change,
            107–110
        Kirkpatrick model, 107–110
        logic model, 106–107, 108f
    Program Sustainability Assessment Tool
        (PSAT), 104, 105b
    quality improvement and long-term
        outcomes, 110
    processes, 110
    structures, 110–111
SWOT (strengths, weaknesses,
    opportunities, threats) analysis,
    54, 56
Systems-based practice (SBP), 3, 20
Systems citizens, 3
Systems citizenship, 36
Systems thinking, 3, 12, 21, 27–30t, 36,
    43, 74

T

Team Assessment Questionnaire and Team
    Performance Observation Tool
    (TAQ-TPOT), 93
Team Climate Inventory (TCI), 93
Team Decision Making Questionnaire
    (TDMQ), 93
Team effectiveness, 12
Team Observed Structured Clinical
    Encounter (TOSCE), 93
Team science, 12
Teamwork Assessment Scale (TAS), 93
Theory-approach logic model, 106
Transformational learning, 40
Transitions of care
    emergency department care and opioid
        use disorder, 58
    hospital discharge and insurance
        barriers, 57
    outpatient appointments and diabetes
        disparities, 57
Triple Aim, 86

U

Undergraduate medical education (UME),
    3, 7, 15, 19, 86
  clinical learning environment, 51–63
  competency recommendations and
    accreditation standards, 22–23t

Undergraduate medical education (UME)
    (Continued)
  program's mission, 113–114
US health care delivery system, 5

V

Value-added educational roles, 45

Value-based care, 27–30t
Value stream mapping, 44–45
Voltage drop, 104

W

Wisely Campaign, 77